Total beauty care, using natural ingredients

NATURAL BEAUTY

Grantown Grammar School

Session ...1986-87...

Class ....S1...........

...Fabrics and Fashion,...
History and Music

PRIZE

awarded to

KAREN HALL

for Merit

Total beauty care, using natural ingredients

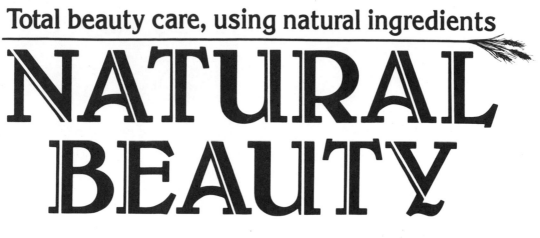

NATURAL BEAUTY

LORNA HORROCKS

with colour illustrations by
MARIANNE YAMAGUCHI

ANGUS
& ROBERTSON
PUBLISHERS

ANGUS & ROBERTSON PUBLISHERS

Unit 4, Eden Park, 31 Waterloo Road,
North Ryde, NSW, Australia 2113, and
16 Golden Square, London W1R 4BN,
United Kingdom

First published in Australia
by Angus & Robertson Publishers in 1980
First published in the United Kingdom
by Angus & Robertson UK in 1981
Reprinted 1987

National Library of Australia
Cataloguing-in-publication data.

Horrocks, Lorna.
  Natural beauty.

  Index
  ISBN 0 207 14420 6

  1. Beauty, Personal. 2. Diet. 3. Food, Natural.
  I. Title.

646.7'2

Typeset in 12 pt Goudy Old Style by Graphicraft Typesetters
Printed in Singapore

CONTENTS

PART VI

FOREWORD

"First we will start with beauty's care
For beauty is the grace of heaven
Well-tended vines productive are,
To well-tilled fields good crops are given;
And so with beauty: but how few
Can show a cheek of perfect hue!"

So wrote the ancient poet Ovid in *The Lover's Handbook*.

For thousands of years people have been looking for ways to care for their skin and improve their appearance. Herbs and other natural ingredients were used in endless combinations to improve the body, the face and the hair — to brighten the eyes, bring colour to the cheeks and improve the spirits. Today we are confronted by a vast range of "beauty care" products manufactured by large companies that advertise heavily and spend much time and effort on packaging, colouring and perfuming their products. But we should not neglect the fascinating heritage we are heirs to, and forget the wisdom of past ages when life was simpler but beauty just as important! The quotations from old herbals and beauty books that you will find scattered throughout this book show just how seriously the business of beauty has always been taken.

This book draws together present-day knowledge with traditional, tried and proven natural ingredients and techniques to give a complete, natural beauty care plan for anyone — man or woman — who takes an interest in his or her appearance. I have given over 140 recipes for cleansers, fresheners, toners, face masks, lotions and creams, for shampoos and conditioners, herbal washes and even herbal teas for relaxing and toning the body. And all of these are free of artificial colour, perfume and preservatives: they are based entirely on natural ingredients. I hope you enjoy trying them — natural beauty care is fascinating and rewarding.

Lorna Horrocks

PART I

FROM THE PAST
TO THE PRESENT

The many quotations I have included in this book will give you a glimpse into the fascinating world of the past. From them it quickly becomes apparent that beauty problems have remained unchanged for thousands of years. People were as concerned in the past as they are today about wrinkles, unwanted body hair, baldness, grey hair, halitosis, sunburn, freckles, acne and pimples, to name a few examples.

In earlier times mostly simple, natural ingredients like honey, oils, fats and herbs were used. Pomades made of perfumed animal and vegetable fats, and unguents or ointments formulated to sweeten, protect and improve the skin and the hair have been with us a long time. Only very recently have the chemical compounds of modern science been offered to us for beauty care.

In the days when all the inhabitants of the earth, mineral, vegetable and animal, were considered equally interesting and valid, some rather strange formulae were accepted which today we find either repulsive or amusing. Three thousand years ago and possibly earlier the Egyptians invented some rather astonishing recipes. From *The Papyrus Ebers* discovered at Thebes in 1862 by Georg Ebers, comes a remedy for "the Eye when something Evil has happened to it" in which the human brain, ground up in various ways, is the main ingredient. We may laugh, but a mere two hundred years ago there were recipes incorporating such unlikely things as dog urine. In the twentieth century, a recipe from "grandmother's day" for the removal of freckles, published in *The News* (South Australia) in 1923, suggested "bullock's blood stirred into alum". Our contemporary knowledge of hygiene prevents us experimenting with some other ancient ideas, for example, re-using the dirty oil scraped off the body at the Roman or Greek bath, or using the water in which the phallus (penis) has been washed, as recommended in an old Egyptian remedy for a mole.

Substances such as lead, mercury, verdigris and arsenic, now known to be very toxic and banned from use, were once incorporated in skin-care recipes. Probably the most widely and generally used of these was lead, and its use continued right up into the nineteenth century, disfiguring the skin, causing baldness, and bringing death to many.

It was not only the ancients who included toxic ingredients in their recipes. Nearer our time, substances later proved to be toxic have been introduced into beauty care. In the late nineteenth century, borax became popular because it easily emulsified beeswax, thus stabilising creams and improving their texture and appearance. The American Medical Association has issued repeated warnings of its possible toxicity following severe poisonings when borax has been ingested or applied topically to broken skin. However, its use continues commercially in cold creams, foundation creams, permanent waving lotions and many others products, while boric acid is used in baby powders, bath powders and mouth washes, to name a few examples. Borax continues to be an ingredient in many so-called natural, home-made beauty recipes.

On the other hand, many harmless and beneficial products such as honey, oils and fats, herbs and spices, grains and meals, milk and vinegar, have been used continuously from prehistoric times to the present day. I find it interesting to think that an ingredient like calamine, a zinc ore, mentioned by Dioscorides in his *Greek Herbal*, has been drying up rashes and pimples for more than two thousand years. Even the "cold cream" which we tend to associate with a modern American firm had its origin in the second century A.D. It is reputed to have been formulated by Galen, a doctor of Greek parentage who practised for many years as physician to the Roman Emperor Marcus Aurelius. Some say he was merely recording a recipe going back to earlier centuries in Greece. The idea of mixing oils and fats with water was a brand new approach and made a different product from those previously used — scented oils and waxes or combinations of ingredients like berries, honey and water, meal, sea-salt and honey, or berries, resins, perfumes and honey.

The cold cream, so-called because evaporation of the water produced a cooling sensation, was more pleasant to apply and more emollient (soothing) to the skin. This recipe became the basis for skin creams throughout the following two thousand years and remains the principle on which today's sophisticated commercial creams are formulated.

We are lucky enough to have been left a fascinating heritage of books giving recommendations and recipes for looking after the body and hair. To quote a few random examples, these include herbals like *The Greek Herbal* by Dioscorides, second century A.D., and *The Complete Herbal* by Nicholas Culpeper, 1653; recipe books like *The Good Housewife's Jewell* by Thomas Dawson, 1596, and *The Housekeeper's Pocketbook* by Sarah Harrison, 1739; health books like *Naturall and Artificial Directions for Health* by William Vaughn, 1600; beauty books like *Delightes for Ladies*, 1602, by Sir Hugh Platt; *Beauties Treasury*, 1705; *The Toilet of Flora*, 1775, a collection of the most simple and approved methods of preparing baths, essences, pomatums; *The Art of Beauty*, 1825, or "the best methods for improving and preserving the shape, carriage and complexion together with the

Theory of Beauty — exercises, diets, home-made toilet preparations";
The Toilet, 1839, a dressing-table companion comprising advice on the
hair, teeth and eyes by the author of *Advice to the Married*; *Toilette*,
1854, or "a guide to the improvement of Personal appearance and the
preservation of health"; *The Art of Beauty*, 1878, by Mrs H.R. Haweis;
The Daily Mirror Beauty Book, 1910. There are numerous books of a
similar kind, giving interesting insights into attitudes to beauty-care
through the ages, recording and passing on many and varied ideas.

Every culture or civilisation and every age has had its
preferences and techniques for looking after the skin and the hair.
Moreover, ideas and ingredients have been exchanged from one
country to another in constant attempts to solve beauty problems and
enhance the appearance. The Egyptians imported from Arabia
ingredients like spikenard, myrrh and frankincense, and they in turn
exported their ideas and their perfumes to the Middle East, to Greece,
and eventually to Rome. This lively exchange continued down the
centuries. For example, the ideas and practices of Europe were given a
boost at the time of the Crusades in the eleventh and twelfth
centuries, when the knights brought home from Asia Minor new
products they had encountered there during the Holy Wars. Possibly
as early as the thirteenth century, individual products like lavender
water and Queen of Hungary water were peddled from one country to
another throughout Europe. Spain became famous for its creams of
vanilla and apricot and its almond paste.

Trade in toiletries, perfumes, dyes and aromatics became more
extensive over the years as more people used beauty aids. From the
Old World, skin-care products and ideas went with colonists to the
New World. Eventually in the twentieth century new developments,
particularly in America, were exported back to Europe, and so the
exchange will go on.

PART II

HEALTH & BEAUTY:
What is Beauty?
Age
Stress & Tension
Sleep

WHAT IS BEAUTY?

The face mirrors to the outside world the state of health and well-being of the body and the mind. That is why we all desire to put forward an attractive face for everyone to see, with a flawless complexion to illustrate that our bodies are healthy and a beautiful expression to manifest the quality of our minds.

It perturbs me how much time is spent talking about disease when people get together to discuss health and beauty. Let us instead be positive in our attitude, because well-being and beauty are interrelated. Beauty is as much in the mind and soul as it is in the physical body. In fact, inner beauty influences outer beauty — through the eyes, facial expression, bodily movement and appearance, tone of voice and the words chosen to give meaning to thoughts.

How can the true potential of each person be brought out?

Everyone can be beautiful, because beauty has many faces. By loving and respecting ourselves, we will take time to look after our bodies, our thoughts will be constructive, and life will cooperate with us, because we are in tune with life.

Envy, fear and insecurity are some of the negative attitudes which can cause poisons to be secreted into the blood from our own glands, undermining the health of our bodies, and destroying the beauty of our faces.

The physical, the mental and the spiritual aspects of each of us must be adequately cared for if we wish to be beautiful. A jar of lotion or cream cannot achieve this on its own. Beauty is a totality of being.

A sensible, healthy diet is the basis of successful beauty care. It shows in the skin, the eyes, the hair and the body and contributes to a general air of well-being. I have discussed diet (and exercise) in detail in Part IV, The Body p. 95.

Herbal teas can help to tone or relax the body, and to prepare it for sleep, and in that way make their own contribution to health and beauty. Below I have given some general instructions in making and using herbal teas. Herbal teas for tonics, relaxation and sleep are listed on pp. 13-20.

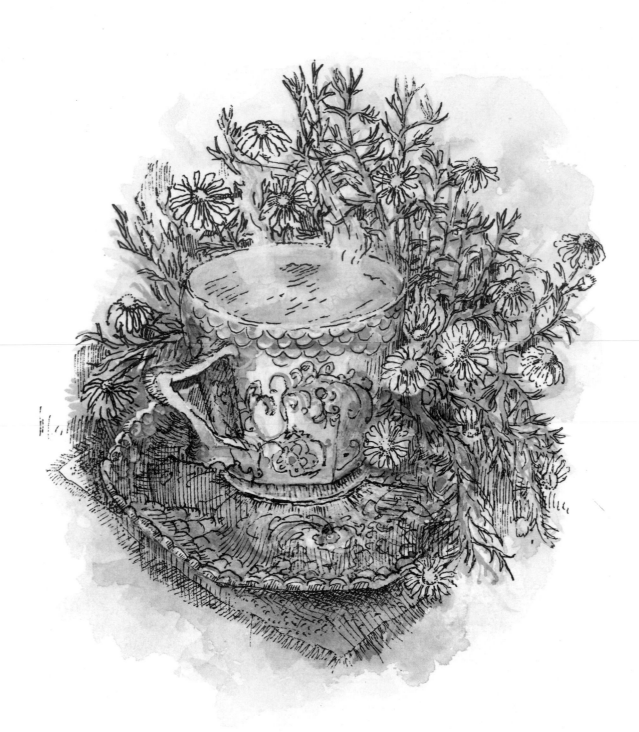

Chamomile tea

✾ Making Herbal Teas: General Instructions

Herbal teas are similar to infusions (p. 39) and may be made with either dried or fresh herbs. As mentioned in the section on making infusions, metal teapots should not be used as they may chemically react with some of the properties of the herbs. Glass, pyrex, china and enamel are suitable. It is generally accepted that one teaspoon of dried herb to one cup of water is an adequate strength for a herbal tea. It is not recommended that milk be added to herbal teas, although honey may be used for sweetening if preferred.

Moderation is the rule when using herbs at home. If, for example, you wish to relax by taking a herbal tea, then a cup in the afternoon or evening is sufficient. You don't use it as you would ordinary tea, drinking numerous cups during the day. Herbs work on the delicate balance of the metabolism and for mild disorders massive doses would not increase the potency of the herbs but more likely cause an imbalance. Medical herbalism is, of course, an entirely different category and should only be practised by a qualified herbalist.

Lettuce cooleth the
heat of the stomacke,

called the heartburning; and it helpeth
it when it is troubled with choler : it
quencheth thirst, and causeth sleepe.

Gerard's Herball
1597

AGE

We are all young. Or to be more precise, we are all as young as we think we are. Society likes to categorise, to put us into convenient little boxes — for example, to divide us into age groups of certain specifications, 25 to 35, or 35 to 45. The implication is that our bodies ought to be at such and such development, our faces should have a certain number of wrinkles and our heads a certain number of grey hairs, and our thoughts ought to run on lines suitable to our age group. What theoretical nonsense!

We are unique beings, individuals, and each and every one of us has something to contribute to life. Age is a state of mind, and many symptoms of old age are more than likely signs of neglect.

There are some people who do not wish to look young. I know a woman with an eighteen-year-old son, who informed me categorically that she wanted some grey hairs and a few wrinkles so that she would look like his mother. The thought of looking the same age as her son made her feel embarrassed and insecure, stripped of her authority. It's all a matter of personality.

What is youth?

Youth is a state of awareness. The younger, the more totally aware. Youth is a time of growth in personality, when of necessity one has to have an open mind to life. But some people are glad to leave youth behind, so they can fit into secure patterns. They don't want to go on growing, experiencing or adapting.

When does youth cease and old age set in? As early as you let it. It can happen in the early twenties. It is not necessarily a question of date of birth.

Through exercise, diet, adequate sleep and the living of a regulated life, that is, one without excesses or extremes, we should remain beautiful, agile and mentally vigorous for many, many years, thus being in a fit state to contribute meaningfully to life around us.

Here are some tonic herbal teas which you may find revitalising when sipped morning or afternoon. Remember not to overdo it, though, drinking cup after cup during the day or continuing to drink a herbal tea over a long period of time. This is unnecessary and, in fact, could be harmful, unbalancing the delicate metabolism.

Tonic Herbal Teas

See p. 11 for general instructions on making herbal teas. Tonic herbs are those which cleanse the body, hence improving its condition. They may be for general purifying or for toning up special organs or glands. Because of your individual metabolism, some herbs will suit you better than others, and only you can judge that.

Herb teas may be sweetened with honey, or blended with other herbs to improve the flavour.

It is a strange quirk of human nature that one ingredient or herb is sought to solve all health problems. Unfortunately this is not possible as health depends on the interaction of so many factors. A miracle herb will never be found. Treat herbal teas with respect and drink them in moderation.

Alfalfa

Alfalfa (lucerne) is a good general tonic which may be eaten raw in salads or its leaves used fresh or dried as a tea. It is rich in vitamins and minerals, and its alkaline properties are particularly valuable for those with a tendency to over-acidity. Use one teaspoon of dried herbs to one cup of boiling water, infused fifteen minutes, to make a tea. Strain and drink.

Basil

This is a nerve tonic as well as a stimulant to the system. Make a tea of the leaves, using one teaspoon of dried herb to one cup of boiling water. Strain and drink.

Borage

Borage is a general blood purifier which encourages the clearing away of toxic residues from the tissues through the bloodstream, and it is also said to imbue the person who drinks it with courage. It is a refreshing tea, taken hot or served cold on a hot day. Use the leaves and some of the blue flowers if you like. Infuse a tablespoon of fresh leaves in a cup of boiling water for fifteen minutes. Strain and drink.

Chickweed

A healing herb, rich in minerals and vitamins, chickweed may be eaten raw in a salad or made into a tea. Infuse a tablespoon of fresh leaves in one cup of boiling water for fifteen minutes. Strain and drink.

Dandelion

A well-known blood-cleansing and tonic herb. The young dandelion leaves may be eaten raw in salad, and are sold commercially for this purpose in Europe and parts of the U.S.A. Make tea by infusing one tablespoon of fresh leaves to a cup of boiling water; or a coffee-type drink by infusing one teaspoon of dried roots in a cup of boiling water. Strain and drink.

Lime or Linden

A very fragrant tea made from the dried flowers is popular in Europe as a refreshing drink. Make the tea by infusing one teaspoon of dried flowers in a cup of boiling water. Strain and drink. Use the flowers a second time if you wish by simmering them gently in fresh water for five minutes.

Nettle

A well-known general tonic and blood purifier, nettle is rich in vitamins and minerals. Use the young shoots fresh or dried to make tea, but if you are picking it fresh, be careful to wear thick protective gloves as it can give you a nasty sting. The dried herb is quite safe to handle. Infuse one teaspoon of dried herb or one tablespoon of fresh herb in a cup of boiling water for ten minutes. Strain and drink.

Purslane

A cooling, tonic herb, rich in vitamins and minerals, purslane may be used fresh in a salad, or the leaves dried for making tea. Infuse one teaspoon of dried herb in one cup of boiling water for ten minutes. Strain and drink.

Rosehip

Rosehips are tonic to the system because of their high content of vitamin C and many minerals. If you want a beautiful complexion, make a tea by soaking six to eight dried hips in a cup of cold water overnight. In the morning, gently bring the water and the hips to the boil and simmer about five minutes. Strain and drink. The same hips may be used once again.

The distilled water of the floures of Rosemary being drunke at morning and evening first and last, taketh away the stench of the mouth and breath, and maketh it very sweet, if there be added thereto, to steep or infuse for certaine daies, a few Cloves, Mace, Cinnamon, and a little Annise seed.

Gerards Herball
1597

STRESS & TENSION

Stress and tension show up drastically in the face, causing tight muscles, grimacing, wrinkles and loss of skin tone. They undermine the health of the body and the mind. Anyone suffering such devastation should do some serious thinking and deliberately rearrange his or her life.

If you suffer from stress and tension, ask yourself some pertinent questions. Do you feel inadequate as a person? Do you accept yourself? Do you trust your own abilities and resources? It is no good avoiding facing your true feelings about yourself, or blaming your inadequacies on anyone else. Only by getting to the basic source of a problem will you solve it satisfactorily. Whether we like it or not, we are all ultimately responsible for our own selves.

It is surprising how much inner strength and talent most people have, given a little appreciation by others. However, human nature being what it is, you won't be appreciated if you don't trust and appreciate yourself. Is your work load too demanding? Are you living beyond your physical or emotional means?

Life should not be a devastating experience; rather a time of joy and fulfilment, but only you can make it that. Take courage. Don't be afraid to say no, to family, friends or the community, when they are asking too much of you.

Are you over-ambitious about acquiring material possessions? If you feel you have to express your worth by a show of material strength, then that is your choice, but be careful that you don't end up finding that your possessions have overwhelmed you or that they have become no more than meaningless clutter in your life.

Are you a hyperactive adult? There are hyperactive adults as well as children, over-stimulated by one or another factor such as wrong diet, overwork, tension. They become adrenalin addicts, turned on by stress, so they tend to seek stress situations, usually without being consciously aware of their problem. It is necessary for each of us to turn off at regular intervals to renew our inner strength.

Today many avenues are being explored to find ways to relax. A variety of answers is being offered from widely differing sources, from medicine to meditation. I can only offer ideas which will perhaps be the first steps to finding what is right for you.

Set aside a little time each day to do nothing. Absolutely nothing. Don't feel guilty. Stare into space, or watch the wind playing in the trees. Turn off. Drink a relaxing cup of herbal tea if it helps (see below).

A simple way to let go is to relax the face. When the face is relaxed, the body tends to follow. Do this by relaxing the lower jaw. Every time you feel your teeth clenching, lips firmly shut, let go. Drop your jaw. It's hard to frown with a relaxed jaw, so you tend to relax your forehead too, and lose those wrinkles across the brow. Another way to relax tense muscles across the forehead is to gently rub in one drop of eucalyptus oil. Be careful, of course, not to get it anywhere near the eyes.

Herbal Teas for Relaxation

See p. 11 for general instructions on making herbal teas.

Lemon Balm

Its flavour is a combination of lemon and tangy mint. Use one teaspoon of dried herbs, or three teaspoons of crushed fresh leaves, to one cup of boiling water. Steep ten minutes and then strain. Sweeten with honey if you wish, but don't add milk. Refreshing taken hot or cold.

Chamomile

This has been used in Europe for many years as a soothing tea. Take one teaspoonful of dried flowerheads to one teacup of boiling water. Infuse five to ten minutes and then strain. Sweeten with honey if you wish. Sip slowly and relax.

Peppermint

Use one teaspoon of dried peppermint leaves to one cup of boiling water. If you have fresh peppermint, then use about three teaspoons of leaves. Infuse ten minutes, then strain and drink.

Catmint

The leaves of the catmint are loved by cats, so if you want to give a feline treat, plant a bush in your garden. To make catmint tea, infuse one teaspoon of dried leaves, and flowers if you have them, to one cup of boiling water. Use three times as much fresh herb if you don't have it dried. Infuse ten minutes, strain and sweeten with honey if you like.

Basil and Borage

Use twice as much borage as basil for this combination tea. For the dried leaves use one teaspoon of borage to half a teaspoon of basil, infused in one cup of boiling water five to ten minutes. For fresh leaves use three times the quantities given for dried. Strain before drinking.

Summer Savory

This is a highly aromatic plant smelling of a mixture of the scents of a summer garden. Steep two teaspoonfuls of the dried leaves, or a handful of fresh leaves, in a cup of boiling water ten minutes. Strain and drink.

Cowslip

You will probably have to grow this delightful herb in your own garden. It is usual to use the flowers dried. Take three teaspoonfuls of flower heads and infuse them in a cup of boiling water for five minutes. Strain and sweeten with honey if desired.

Lemon Verbena

The strongly perfumed leaves of this shrub make a lemon-flavoured tea which is sedative in effect. Taken in the hot weather it is very cooling. Cut up half a dozen leaves, which is equivalent to about two teaspoonfuls. Pour over one cup of boiling water, steep five minutes, then strain and drink.

SLEEP

To retire each night in peace is everyone's ideal. We all need regular, restful, natural sleep to keep healthy and it is a great enhancer of the complexion.

Supposing you can't sleep? Ask yourself a few searching questions. Are you overworking every day? Do you feel almost too exhausted to get ready for bed? Then it is no wonder you are restless at night, because you are creating a vicious circle of overtiredness. Overtiredness from the day leads to an inability to relax and regenerate at night, which causes more fatigue the next day. Break out of this abnormal rhythm by re-examining your daytime activities.

If you are not overworking, and feel your daily habits are not creating excessive fatigue, yet cannot sleep restfully at night, look to your bedding and sleeping habits. Is your bed comfortable? Does it sag in the middle? Do you sleep clinging to the side of a hill on one side of the double bed? Try twin beds. Is the mattress rock hard? Are your bedclothes too heavy? A continental feather quilt in the winter is an ideal solution to this problem.

Do you get sufficient fresh air at night? You'll feel jaded in the morning if you don't. Besides, stuffy, dry rooms dehydrate the skin and can cause an accumulation of fluid around the eyes, making them baggy in the mornings.

Is your sleeping posture restful? Lie on your side to rest your spine, but don't lean the weight of your body on your face. A sprawling posture in bed distorts the spine, the face and the neck.

Is your diet adequate? Are you getting sufficient vitamins and minerals to soothe the nervous system and tone it up? Calcium and magnesium intakes are often below required levels.

Herbal teas which are soothing and strengthening to the nerves (nervines) may be taken at bedtime to help promote restful sleep if you are having problems with insomnia.

Herbal Teas to Promote Sleep

See p. 11 for general instructions on making herbal teas.

Hops

Hops have been known for many years to promote a restful night's sleep. To make a bedtime tea, place two teaspoonfuls of hops in one cup of cold water, heat and simmer two minutes, strain and drink.

Lavender

Use either the flowers or the leaves to make a tea. Infuse one teaspoon of flowers or two teaspoons of leaves to one cup of boiling water for ten minutes before straining. Add the flowers to other herbs, such as scented geranium leaf or comfrey leaves, if you wish to vary the flavour.

Red Clover

Either infuse two teaspoons of flowers in one cup of boiling water for ten to fifteen minutes, then strain, or simmer one teaspoon of flowers for five minutes in one cup of water, then strain. A blood cleanser, which encourages the clearing away of toxic residues from the tissues through the bloodstream, as well as being soothing to the nerves.

Lettuce

Use fresh lettuce leaves, but choose the dark green outside leaves of the garden lettuce, or better still, grow small loose-leaf (cos or mignonette) lettuces. Simmer gently one smallish lettuce in two cups of water, for ten to fifteen minutes. Strain and drink.

Aniseed

Crush one teaspoon of seed, then infuse it in one cup of boiling water for ten minutes. Strain and drink. Delightfully aromatic. It may also be made with milk.

Elderflower

Either infuse one cup of fresh flowers in one cup of boiling water for ten minutes and then strain, or use one teaspoon dried flowers to one cup of boiling water, infuse five minutes, then strain and sweeten with honey.

Rhodides. Pomanders of Roses

Pomanders of Roses, which they call
Rhodides, are made after this fashion.
Of fresh Roses, which beginne to fade,
before they have taken any wett,
dragms 40: of Indian Nard, ten
dragms, of Myrrh six dragms. These
being beaten small are made into
little balls, of the weight of three Oboli,
and they are dried in the shade, and
layd vp in vase fictili non picato, close
stopped round about. Somme adde
also of Costus 2 dragms, & as much
of Illyrick Iris, mixing also Chian
wine with Hony. The use of it is to be put
about women's necks instead of necklaces,
dulling the unsavourie smell of the
sweat. They vse the same also being
beaten small in medicines made to
represse the sweat, & in ointments to
anoint withall after bathing, & being
dried in, they are washed off with
cold water.

Dioscorides A.D. 60

A Bag to
Smell Unto for Melancholy,
or to Cause one to Sleep:

Take drie Rose leaves, keep them close
in a glasse which will keep them sweet,
then take powder of mints, powder of
Cloves in a grosse powder, and put
the same to the Rose leaves, then put all
these together in a bag, and take that
to bed with you, and it will cause you
to sleep, and it is good to smell unto
at other times.

'Ram's Little Dadoen' 1606
Quoted in E.S. Rohde
'A Garden of Herbs'

Herb Pillows

Herb pillows have been used for centuries as a type of aromatherapy. They are usually made as a small pillow or sachet of herbs to be put in the pillowcase with the regular sleeping pillow, or placed underneath it. Dried herbs are always used for this purpose.

The types of herbs chosen are those which are known to have a calming or sedative effect on the body and mind. Hops are probably best known for use in a sleep pillow, so they could be used as a base with the addition of other herbs. Choose from peppermint, sage, lemon balm, lavender, catmint, clover, bay leaf, cowslip, chamomile, lemon verbena, lemon thyme, mother of thyme, marjoram. Add a few cloves, pine needles or lemon or orange peel to vary the fragrance. In fact, you can use any combination of herbs which appeals to your olfactory senses.

To make the pillow, simply sew up a bag from two pieces of cloth and fill it with herbs. It can be whatever size you prefer, ranging from 15 cm × 10 cm (6 in × 4 in) to 30 cm (12 in) square.

PART III

THE FACE:
The Skin
The Eyes
The Neck
The Lips
The Teeth

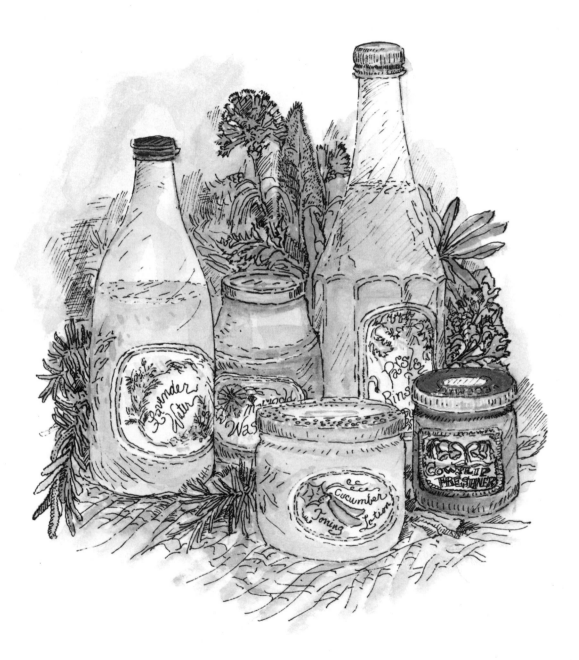

Ninon de L'Enclos
Ointment

Oil of Almonds	4 ozs
Hogs Lard	3 ozs
Spermaceti	1 oz

Melt, and add 3 fluid ounces of
expressed juice of houseleek, and
stir till cool. Scent with a few
drops of esprit de rose.

C. F. Leyel
'The Magic of Herbs'

THE SKIN

The foundation of a healthy beautiful skin is diet. I have mentioned the general principles in the section on diet on page 135, but I wish to be more specific here because there are aspects of diet which bear directly on the condition of the skin. Are you getting sufficient polyunsaturated fats? These are essential to a healthy skin and do not cause facial oiliness. They are found in cereal grains, nuts and cold-pressed nut and vegetable oils.

Plenty of vitamin C is fundamental to a beautiful skin, because it builds collagen and elastin, the bonding and structural substances which give tone and resilience. There is no need to resort to tablets. Eat bean sprouts, green and red peppers, blackcurrants, oranges and lemons. Then there are guavas and rosehips, so your diet need not be restricted or dull. There is infinite variety to suit every palate.

Lack of vitamin A can cause dryness of the skin. Eat dandelion, parsley, watercress, carrots, pumpkins, celeriac.

If your skin is unbalanced, either flaky or too oily, or if your lips peel, then check your intake of vitamin B foods. Oats, yeast, bran, goat's milk, whole rice, sunflower seeds, sprouted seeds and grains are some of the sources.

Skin Types

Normal skin

Normal skin is smooth, finely-textured, soft and supple. If you are lucky enough to possess this skin type, treasure it by using light cleansers and lotions and mild toners and fresheners.

Dry skin

Dry skin is usually thin and delicate and often flaky and prone to fine lines. It sometimes feels tighter than it should. Extremely rich and greasy creams are not good for it because they strangulate the pores, often enlarging them and so creating an extra problem. Use light oils and lotions for moisturising and choose herbal toners which are mild and not too astringent. Try to restore the pH or acid-alkali balance with the application of such things as cucumber juice or diluted vinegar so that the sebaceous glands are encouraged to function.

Generally speaking, the emollient and hydrating herbs (chamomile, comfrey, cowslip, elderflower, fennel, marshmallow, orange blossom, rose, violet) are the best to use in lotions and toners for dry skin. But there is no hard and fast rule. Astringent herbs can be good for dry skins, for example, if blended with emollient herbs or oils and gels, and many herbs are suitable for all skin types (see herb chart, p. 168). If the skin is sensitive as well as dry, see the notes on sensitive skin below.

Oily skin

Oily skin is shiny and coarser-textured, often with enlarged pores. It is prone to blackheads and spots. Don't use alcohol to reduce the oiliness of the skin, as it will only worsen the problem. Many herbal toners are suitable for reducing oiliness and tightening the pores (see list of suitable herbs below). Egg-white makes a nice mild face-mask. Don't overdry the skin; moisturise with a light lotion. Aim to restore your skin's acid-alkali balance so that the sebaceous glands cease to produce such large amounts of oil.

Astringent and cleansing herbs are generally the best to choose when treating an oily skin. These are: cinquefoil, clary sage, comfrey, cucumber, dandelion, horsetail, houseleek, hyssop, lavender, lemon balm, lemongrass, lemon verbena, marigold, mint, parsley, sage, wych hazel and yarrow. But don't forget that many herbs are suited to all skin types (see herb chart, p. 168) and that many of the strengthening and anti-inflammatory herbs (chamomile, cowslip, fennel, lettuce, elderflower, orange blossom, rose, violet) are suitable for oily skins.

Combination skin

The person with this skin type will have to follow two beauty routines, one for the dry areas, and another for the oily. I think the oily areas balance up more easily in this type of skin than when the whole face is oily, so don't despair.

Sensitive skin

This skin is usually fine-textured and often prone to reddish veins and

Remedy to Beautify
the Skin.

Meal - of - Alabaster
Meal - of - Natron
Sea - salt
Honey
Mix into one in this Honey and
anoint the body therewith.

'The Papyrus Ebers'
1500 B.C.

Yellow Complexion

Persons suffering from this should never wash the face with soap; always use an oatmeal bag and you must attend to your general health. A yellow skin is usually the sign of biliousness or some other derangement of the liver, and one should be careful of their diet and avoid constipation.

This preparation will be found very valuable to persons suffering from the above, and if used for one month, the sallowness should be removed.

4oz pure lard, 1oz Elderberry Flowers, 1 tablespoonful Vinegar, Camphor the size of a nutmeg, 1oz Almond oil, 1oz Eau de Cologne, 1oz Lavender Water.

Massage gently into the skin.

'Madame Cristo's Beauty Guide'
1923

patches. Keep to light oils and lotions for cleansing and moisturising, and mild herbal toners and compresses to soothe the skin and reduce redness and veins. It is usually wise for people with sensitive skins to stay away from the stimulating herbs (lavender, limeflower, mint, nettle, sage, southernwood, summer savory, thyme).

❋ *Dull skin*

Dull skin has lost the bloom of vitality and the soft glow of renewal. It looks matt and lifeless. Its acid balance has slipped. If it is oily or large-pored skin use diluted cider vinegar or lemon juice, or cucumber juice to balance it. If it is dry skin, use buttermilk or cucumber juice.

❋ *Mature skin*

Older skin can be toned and softened and restored to much of its former beauty. The skin is a wonderfully regenerating organ, given encouragement. Use a light hand with makeup if you must use it, as this dries and ages the skin.

A Skin-care Routine

The basic procedures for a beneficial skin-care routine follow three logical steps: cleanse; tone; moisturise.

But, please, don't overdo it. *Moderation* is the rule. Your facial skin is a living, breathing, eliminating and self-regenerating organ, so give it a chance. Over-cleansing, harsh toning, or clogging the pores with lashings of nourishing cream will not achieve the desired results.

Moreover, don't use just one type of cleanser, one toner, and one moisturising lotion day in, day out, year after year. Give your skin a change. Become observant of its requirements, which alter from time to time, according to climate, diet or health. Skin can also become sensitised to a particular ingredient.

Be gentle when applying preparations to your face. Don't irritate or drag on the skin. Lotions should be smoothed on, then any excess blotted off after about fifteen minutes.

Extreme heat or cold is bad for the skin, so a facial sauna or putting the face under an ice-cold shower in the mornings is not recommended.

If you look after your skin correctly, clean it regularly, and don't clog up the pores with makeup or heavy, rich creams, there will be no necessity to deep cleanse it with steam. Only in exceptional circumstances, such as the presence of many stubborn blackheads or pimples, should the face be subjected to steaming. Sensitive skin should never be steamed. Tepid or blood heat is the correct temperature for anything applied to the skin.

Every person must work out his or her own routine to suit individual needs and skin type, as well as the physical environment in which he or she lives.

A dry climate with low rainfall, whether hot or cold, is very dehydrating. Air-conditioning in summer and artificially heated rooms in winter are equally drying. It is easy to overlook the fact that the skin dehydrates as much in the winter as the summer, so we should not be careless about looking after ourselves when the cold weather comes.

The following are guidelines to help in the formulation of a personal routine.

1. Cleansing

This should be done once a day, preferably at night when the buildup of dirt is heaviest. People with very oily skins will need to cleanse again in the morning, as oil attracts dirt which adheres to it. Recipes for herbal cleansers may be found on pp. 41-9.

2. Toning

Toning means wiping over with a herbal liquid to keep the skin firm and fine in texture, thus counteracting any tendency to large pores or sagging and wrinkling of the skin. Regular toning is important to the skin. Do it whenever you feel it is necessary. Toning has traditionally followed cleansing, but this depends entirely on how one has cleansed, and what manner of cleanser has been used.

An oily or thick cream cleanser merely wiped off with tissues would certainly necessitate toning the skin to remove excessive oiliness and to correct the drag effect which heavier oils and creams have on the skin.

If one uses a light cleanser, or an oily cleanser removed with cotton wool pads thoroughly moistened in a herbal infusion, followed by a dry towelling, there will be no need to tone. The skin will already be soft yet firm in texture.

Recipes for herbal toners may be found on pp. 53-5.

3. *Moisturising*

A tradition throughout the cosmetic world has long been the "nourishing night cream". In my personal experience and observation, this is not the correct way to improve the skin. At night, the skin needs to be as free as possible to breathe and repair itself. All it needs is a light oil or lotion to prevent dehydration, and the oil blotted before going to bed to remove the excess, leaving a light, scarcely visible film on the skin. Lotions are usually satisfactory if allowed to dry on the skin.

If you must use a cream, moisturising should be done in the morning, as that is when the skin needs protection and a boost to cope with the extra wear and tear of the daytime. However, in most cases a lotion would be quite adequate. During the day use any of the lotions you prefer, applying when you feel it is necessary. They will give a certain toning effect as well as maintaining softness.

Recipes for herbal moisturisers may be found on pp. 59-74.

Recipes for Cleansers, Toners, Masks & Lotions

About the Recipes and How to Make Them

I have tried to keep the recipes for all my facial applications and other things as pure and simple as possible — consequently they may not look like the commercial products you are probably used to.

In herbal preparations, the colours tend to be plain, even dingy, but to add colour is to sacrifice purity to superficial appearance. You may wish to add a drop of essential oil to improve the smell of some of the lotions, but I prefer to use them unperfumed.

I do not use chemical additives (for example, emulsifiers like borax or triethanalomine), to ensure that no changes are made to the essential qualities of the herbs.

Preservatives are not used except for the occasional drop of tincture of benzoin. If you wish to take your own lotions with you when travelling this will keep them fairly well for two to three weeks.

Waxes and sticky unguents I keep to a minimum as I feel that they merely sit on the surface of the skin, often dragging and stretching it and strangulating the pores.

It is essential to "try out" various lotions because we all have different skin reactions. Although all the components are pure and simple, it is always possible that a person may be sensitive to one or another of them. It is up to you to find out which of the recipes suit your particular skin type and metabolism. Should you already know that your skin reacts badly to any specific ingredient, then of course avoid recipes which use it.

To make these cosmetic recipes you will require only very simple equipment. Measurements are given in teaspoons and tablespoons. Generally speaking, four teaspoons are equal to one tablespoon in liquid measure. It doesn't matter if they are a little smaller or larger than the spoons I used — providing you keep to the same teaspoon as a measure in your recipe, everything will be in the correct proportions.

I save up all the small screw-top jars that come my way for storing the lotions. To make sure they are washed thoroughly, I put them through the dishwasher or boil them as the extra heat in the water removes all odours. Special screw-top jars may be purchased from a chemist if you prefer.

Adequately label everything you make, because the memory can be very short at times, and you don't want your favourite lotion ending up as the salad dressing!

When it is necessary to use heat in the preparation, stand a jar in a saucepan of hot water and place the ingredients inside the jar to melt before pouring into your storage jar.

You may wish to use a blender to homogenise the ingredients, but a good shaking by hand is usually sufficient. A mortar and pestle are useful if you need to grind up herbs or bruise them before use. Always use a wooden spoon if it is necessary to stir, particularly when heating any ingredients.

Before you begin on the interesting task of making and trying out the recipes, I should like to point out that there is no such thing as the magic lotion which will change your skin condition overnight. Time and perseverance are necessary to achieve results.

Ingredients

If an ingredient or term is unfamiliar to you, look it up in the ABC of ingredients starting on p. 167. I have given simple information on every ingredient used there.

Distilled water should be used in all recipes, as tap water contains chemicals and impurities which may interfere with the action of the herbs and other ingredients. Rainwater is not really pure, but can substitute.

1 part Friar's Balsam
20 parts Rosewater

Shake well and apply to face as often
as possible.
   I might mention this is a splendid
lotion for nearly all complexion troubles,
and is the same as a very expensive
patent preparation to which a
fanciful name has been given.

'Madame Cristo's Beauty Guide'
1923

The Original Cold Cream

Melt one part of purified or white wax in four parts of rose oil (olive oil in which rose petals have been macerated). Pour the melted liquid from one vessel to another adding a little cold water each time. (Some say a little vinegar or spirits of vinegar were added).

Galen 131-201 A.D.
'Methodus Medendi vel de Morbis Curandis'

Many of the recipes list as ingredients herbal infusions or decoctions, or gels. General instructions for making these are given below. Mostly the quantities required for the recipes are small, and you may have some infusion, decoction or gel over. Look up your "leftover" by name (e.g. lavender infusion) in the index at the back of the book to find out in which other recipes it appears or to which other uses it can be put.

Keeping Herbal Preparations

In these recipes I give only very small quantities, so you can make up a small amount of a lotion to try on your skin and thus avoid wastage if it is not suitable. Another vital reason for this is to keep all applications as fresh as possible. Being organic, they will deteriorate, some more quickly than others, depending on the ingredients. Should you like a lotion or cream then by all means make up a large amount, but be sure to refrigerate it, particularly in the summer. Always pour preparations out of the container onto your palm, or take a little out with a clean spoon, rather than plunging the fingers into them and introducing bacteria which may cause deterioration.

Simple herbal infusions and fresheners, where the herb has been merely steeped in water, will not keep for more than a few days without refrigeration, unless the weather is cold. Naturally there are exceptions such as lavender which is very antiseptic and consequently has good keeping qualities. If commercial wych hazel or an alcohol such as gin or brandy, or a few drops of benzoin tincture is added to an infusion it will keep quite well in a cupboard. The lotions and creams made with lemon juice and the gels (particularly quince gel) keep for several weeks in a cool dark cupboard.

Infusions, gels, lotions and creams will keep for several months in the refrigerator, providing their containers are spotlessly clean. I have kept orange flower water, rosewater; marigold, fennel and elderflower infusions and quince gel in the refrigerator for six months without their spoiling.

How to Make Herbal Infusions

An infusion is similar to a tea. You make it by pouring boiling water over a herb and allowing it to steep to extract its active ingredients. Always cover the infusing herb with a lid to minimise loss of volatile elements through steam evaporation.

Do not use metal teapots to make infusions, as they may chemically react with some of the properties of the herb. Glass, pyrex, china and enamel are suitable.

Fresh herbs must be used at at least twice the quantity of dried herbs for an equivalent strength infusion.

Exact quantities are not absolutely crucial in herbal preparations. Besides, herbs differ according to location, soil and method of drying. The standard brew is 30g of dried herb to 500 ml water (1 oz to 1 pint). A mild infusion is 15 g to 500 ml (½ oz to 1 pint), and a weak infusion is 5 g to 500 ml (¼ oz to 1 pint). Herbs vary according to the density of material, so roots are very often heavier than leaves, while flowers may be much lighter. Consequently, it is difficult to give a general measure in cups and tablespoons to suit every herb. However, taking one cup of herb as being approximately 30 g (1 oz), I have given three average strengths of infusion as a quick reference.

Standard — three level tablespoons to one cup of water
Mild   — one and a half level tablespoons to one cup of water
Weak   — half a level tablespoon to one cup of water

Mild or weak infusions are usually sufficiently strong for cosmetic purposes, but this is only a guide; vary them as you wish.

Use herbs suited to your skin type (pp. 30-3, 166).

Herbal Decoctions

A decoction is where the herb is gently boiled in water to extract the active ingredients. The harder parts of the plants, such as roots, bark or seeds, are usually treated in this way. A non-metal container should be used.

How to Make Gels

Arrowroot Gel

To make arrowroot gel, combine one teaspoon of powdered arrowroot with four tablespoons of water and heat gently, stirring continuously until the mixture thickens and clears. Remove from heat.

Irish Moss Gel

Soak 30 g (1 oz) Irish moss in 500 ml (1 pint) of water overnight in a non-metal container. Next day, slowly bring to the boil, then drain.

Quince Gel

Take about twenty-five seeds from ripened quinces and put them in a non-metal container with 250 ml (½ pint) cold rainwater or distilled water. Bring slowly to the boil and simmer gently about fifteen minutes. Stir to prevent seeds sticking. The mixture will thicken to a gel. Strain off the seeds and keep them in the refrigerator to use several times.

How to apply lotions

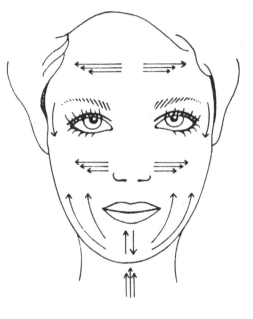

These movements create the least drag on the skin.

Cleansers

Quick Cleansers

Almond milk (p. 54) for oily skin; apricot oil or any cold-pressed vegetable oil, for dry skin; buttermilk, for any skin type.
    Apply to the face with saturated cottonwool. Rub gently with the fingertips to loosen dirt, then wipe with soft tissues.

Herbal Cleansing Infusions

Make a mild-strength infusion of a herb suitable to your skin type (pp. 30-3). Apply to your face with cottonwool and wipe dry with a soft towel.

Oatmeal Cleanser
For any skin type.

1 tablespoon oatmeal
2 tablespoons quince or Irish moss gel
(p. 40-1)
1 tablespoon standard herbal infusion (p. 39)
Herbs suitable for the infusion are elderflower, fennel, lavender (not for sensitive skin) or marigold. To make fennel seed infusion, pour one cup boiling water over one tablespoon crushed seed and steep until cold.

Mix the ingredients to a paste.

Rub over the face and neck. Leave two minutes, then rinse off.

Honey Cleansing Lotion
For any skin type.

1 teaspoon honey
2 tablespoons warm milk
Blend together to make a thin lotion.

Rub over the face and neck with the fingertips. Rinse off.

Fennel Cleansing Lotion
For any skin type.

1 teaspoon fennel seed infusion (see below)
1 teaspoon honey
2 tablespoons buttermilk
To make a fennel seed infusion, pour one cup of boiling water over one tablespoon of crushed seed and steep until cool. Mix ingredients together.

Smooth the lotion over the face and neck to cleanse, rubbing gently. Wipe off with cottonwool dipped in fennel seed infusion. Pat dry.

Sage Cleansing Lotion
For all types except sensitive skin.

1 teaspoon olive oil
1 teaspoon honey
1 drop cider vinegar
2 teaspoons standard sage infusion (p. 39)

Combine the oil and honey, warming a little. Add the sage infusion and the vinegar. Stir well.

Buttermilk and Honey Cleansing Lotion
For any skin type.

2 teaspoons buttermilk
1 teaspoon honey
1 teaspoon almond oil
1 teaspoon apricot oil
2 teaspoons standard marigold infusion (p. 39)

Note: when making marigold infusion, steep until cold.

Combine ingredients in a small glass jar with a lid and shake well before using.

Gently rub over the face and neck and leave ten minutes. Wash off with rainwater, distilled water or a mild herbal infusion (p. 39) made from elderflower, lemongrass or fennel. A lovely summertime cleanser.

On a hot, trying day, for a pick-me-up, wash off with a facial freshener such as five tablespoons of water mixed with one teaspoon of fresh lemon juice.

Non-Oily Cleansing Lotion

1 tablespoon quince or Irish moss gel (p. 40-1)
1 teaspoon mild herbal infusion suitable to skin type (p. 39)

Combine ingredients and shake thoroughly.

For a deep pore cleanser, add half a teaspoon of honey.

Mint Cleanser
For stimulating the skin.

2 teaspoons coconut oil
1 teaspoon standard mint infusion (p. 39)
1 drop cider vinegar

Melt the coconut oil, add the mint and vinegar. Shake.

A cleanser which leaves the skin soft and refreshed.

Bran Deep-Pore Cleanser
For dry skin.

1 tablespoon quince or Irish moss gel (p. 40-1)
½ tablespoon olive oil
1 tablespoon bran

Combine ingredients.

This is rather crumbly on application, but very cleansing and toning. Rub over the face and neck. Leave two minutes, then rinse off thoroughly with a mild chamomile infusion (p. 39).

Olive Oil Cleanser
Good for removing city grime. For any skin type.

2 teaspoons olive oil
1 teaspoon honey

Mix together.

Apply to the face and neck, rubbing in with the fingertips. Wash off with a mild chamomile infusion (p. 39). It may be necessary to warm the oil and honey a little in cold weather as the honey tends to become rather granular.

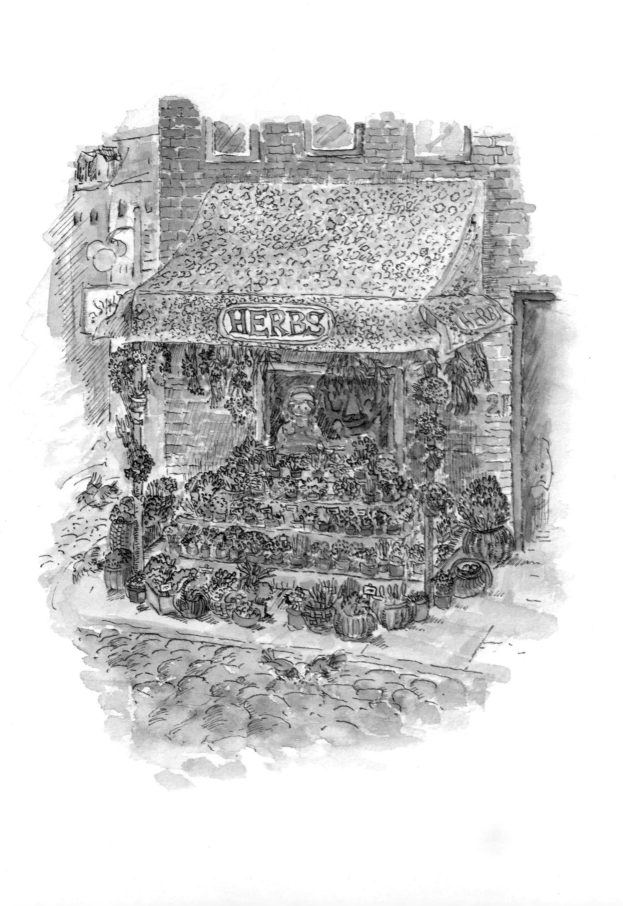

Wild Olive Oil

But ye oyle which is of the wild olive
is more binding & the second in use
for ye state of health. It is convenient
instead of Rosaceum for ye Caput
dolentibus, stays sweatings, & the haire
falling. It doth cleanse Furfures, &
Ulcera capitas manantia, & Scabiem,
& Lepras, & it keeps off gray haires
a long tyme from them which are
anointed therewith dayly.

Dioscorides A.D. 60.

Olive-oil has the property of imparting warmth to the body and protecting it against the cold, and also that of cooling the head when heated.
Those parents of all the vices, the Greeks, have diverted the use of olive-oil to serve the purpose of luxury by making it a regular practice in their gymnasiums; the governors of those institutions have been known to sell the scrapings of the oil for 80,000 sesterces.

PLINY - the Elder
A.D. 23 - 79

'Natural History'

Rose Cold Cream

Almond oil	1lb
Rose Water	1lb
White Wax ⎫ each Spermaceti ⎭	1oz
Otto of Roses	Half dram

C. F. Leyel

'The Magic of Herbs' 1926

Thyme Cleanser
For oily or disturbed skin.

1 tablespoon milk
1 heaped teaspoon wheatmeal flour
1 level teaspoon cornflour
2 tablespoons standard thyme infusion (p. 39)
Put the milk, flour, and cornflour into a glass jar standing in hot water, and stir until it begins to thicken. Add the thyme infusion and stir in well. Allow to cool.

Lemon Cleansing Cream
For all types except sensitive skin.

1 teaspoon anhydrous lanolin (wool fat)
½ teaspoon lemon juice
2 teaspoons olive oil
1 teaspoon almond oil
Combine ingredients in a small glass or china container and stir thoroughly.

Apply to face and neck as a cleanser and wipe off with a mild elderflower infusion (p. 39). Leaves the skin soft and clean.

Lemon Balm and Verbena Cleansing Cream
For all types except sensitive skin.

2 teaspoons unsalted butter
2 teaspoons olive oil
1 teaspoon mild lemon balm infusion (p. 39)
1 teaspoon mild lemon verbena infusion
(p. 39)
½ teaspoon lemon juice

Soften the butter and stir in the oil. Add the herbal infusions and the lemon juice and stir thoroughly. Rub the cream over the face to loosen dirt, then wash off with wet cottonwool.

Fresheners

Elderflower Freshener
For any skin type.

Make a mild infusion of elderflowers (p. 39). Strain through
cheesecloth into a bottle. Add one or two drops of tincture of benzoin
to one cup of infusion.

Fennel Freshener
For any skin type.

Make an infusion of fennel seed by pouring one cup of boiling water
over one tablespoon of crushed seed. Steep until cold. Strain and
bottle.
        For a variation combine equal quantities of chamomile and
fennel infusions.

Violet Freshener
For any skin type.

Simmer one tablespoon of chopped violet flowers in one cup of water
for about two minutes, then steep until cold. Strain and bottle.

Cowslip Freshener
For any skin type.

Infuse three teaspoons of dried flowers in 150 ml (¼ pint) boiling water
for five minutes. Strain and bottle.

Parsley Freshener
For disturbed skin.

Make a standard infusion (p. 39) of fresh parsley leaves. Steep fifteen
minutes then strain and bottle.

Eau-de-Cologne Mint Freshener
For oily skin.

Chop up and bruise two tablespoons of fresh mint leaves. Infuse in
one cup of boiling water, allowing to steep until cold. Strain and
bottle.

Face Lotion

4 tablespoons Elderflower water

½ teaspoon Benzoin (added drop by
                drop, stirring constantly)

5 drops Glycerine

5 drops tincture of Myrrh

My Great-Grandmother's recipe
                circa 1910

Chamomile Freshener
For any skin type.

Make a mild infusion of chamomile flowers (p. 39). Strain and bottle.

Lavender Water
For oily skin.

Pour one cup of boiling water over one teaspoon of dried lavender
flowers and allow to steep until cold. Strain and bottle.

Rose Petal Skin Freshener
‘For oily skin.

½ cup rose petal infusion (see below)
2 tablespoons wych hazel
1 teaspoon rosewater (from the chemist)

To make rose petal infusion, take the petals of one dark red, strongly scented rose, or one of the old-fashioned herbal roses, and pour over half a cup of boiling distilled water. Leave to infuse for several hours in a covered container. Strain the infusion into a bottle, then add the wych hazel and rosewater. Shake.

Limeflower (Linden) Skin Stimulant
To stimulate circulation in the skin.

1 tablespoon dried limeflowers
1 cup distilled water

Infuse the flowers in boiling water for ten minutes, then strain and stand to cool.

Apply to the face and neck. Leave on fifteen minutes, then rinse off with tepid water. The mucilaginous properties of limeflowers leave the skin soft.

Snapdragon

Antirrhinon, which some
call Anarrhinon & some have
called it Lychnis agrestis, is a
herb like to Anagallis in ye leaves &
ye stalk, but ye flowers are purple, like
Leucoion, but lesser, whence also it was
called sylvestris Lychnis. But it bears a fruit like
ye nostrils of a calf, carnation like in appearance.
But it is storied that this is opposite to poisons,
being hanged about one, & that it makes
one fair, being annointed on with
lilly-oil, or Cyprine.

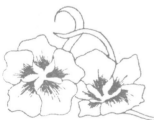

Dioscorides

A.D. 60

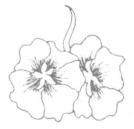

Cucumber lotion for
the skin is excellent in
this severe weather, and much
recommended for people
whose faces and hands chap
in the cold wind.

"PAM"

June 1923

✿ *Toners*

Cucumber Toning Lotion
For any skin type.

The cucumber has long been used as a beauty aid, particularly for oily skins. However, its toning and soothing qualities can be equally valuable for those with dry or sensitive skins. After you have been using emollients and oils, or lotions containing these, use cucumber lotion as a combined cleanser and toner.

Take a cucumber, organically-grown and free of pesticides, if possible, wash it thoroughly, then put it through the juice extractor, skin and all. If peeled and only the white flesh used the cucumber seems to lose some of its natural balance and is too astringent.

Wipe the green liquid over the face and neck to cleanse, cool and tone, and leave to dry on the skin. It is not necessary to wash off this liquid, in fact to do so would negate its effect. Just leave it alone as a treatment until you wish to cleanse or moisturise. This reduces facial shine, often a problem of thin, sensitive skins, and tightens up lines and wrinkles, including those under the eyes.

Honey Toning Lotion
For any skin type.

Mix half a teaspoon of honey with one tablespoon of warmed, distilled water. Apply to face and neck and leave to dry on for half an hour. Gently rinse off and pat dry.

Buttermilk Toner
For any skin type.

Smooth buttermilk over the face and neck, and allow to dry on ten to fifteen minutes. This is gently astringent and restores the acid mantle to the skin. Rinse off with tepid water and blot dry.

Comfrey Root Toning Night Lotion
For any skin type.

Take one piece of comfrey root about the size of your little finger. Scrub off the brown outside skin with a pot mitt. Place the clean root in a non-metal container, such as a pyrex coffee pot, with one cup of rainwater or distilled water. Simmer twenty minutes, allow to cool, then strain and bottle.

After cleansing the face and neck and wiping dry, apply the comfrey lotion and allow to dry on the skin. Leave overnight.

Gentle Quince Toner
For dry skin.

Smooth a small amount of quince gel (p. 41) over the face and neck. This may be left on for as long as you like.

Almond Milk Toning Lotion
A toning, yet softening lotion
for all skin types.

2 tablespoons almond meal
150 ml (¼ pint) distilled water
Place in a blender and whip two minutes. Strain through cheesecloth and bottle. Apply to the face daily and leave to dry on the skin. It is not necessary to wash off this liquid, in fact to do so would negate its effect. Just leave it alone as a treatment until you wish to cleanse or moisturise.

Violet Leaf Toning Lotion
For any skin type.

1 egg white
1 teaspoon honey
½ teaspoon almond oil
3 teaspoons violet leaf juice (see below)
To make violet leaf juice, simply put a large handful of violet leaves through the juice extractor. Beat the egg white. Add the honey, oil and violet juice, beating them in. A blender is useful for this recipe. Store in a glass jar with a screw top. Apply to the face daily, leaving on as long as you prefer. Rinse off gently and blot dry.

Horsetail Skin Tonic
For normal to oily skin.

2 tablespoons horsetail infusion (see below)
1 teaspoon oatmeal gruel (see below)
To make horsetail infusion, soak two teaspoons of horsetail in one cup of boiling water overnight. To make oatmeal gruel, boil two tablespoons of steel-cut oats in a small cup of water for five minutes. Strain off the gruel water to use. Combine ingredients in a glass bottle, screw on lid and shake.

Apply to the face morning or night and leave on as long as you prefer. Rinse off with tepid water and pat dry.

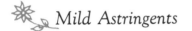 *Mild Astringents*

Astringent for any type of skin

1 teaspoon cider vinegar
2 tablespoons distilled water
Mix together.

Astringent for oily skin

1 teaspoon lemon juice
2 tablespoons distilled water
Mix together.

✾⚘ *Masks*

The need to use a face mask won't arise so often if you keep your skin cleaned and toned on a daily basis. People with dry skins should use only mild tightening masks, thickened with arrowroot, bran, steel-cut oats gruel or egg white. Those with oily skin and large pores will probably want something firmer, so use yoghurt, oatmeal flour or kaolin powder as a binder.

Apply a mask to a clean skin, staying well clear of the sensitive areas of the face, around the eyes and the lips. Leave it on until it has completely set, then wash off thoroughly with tepid water. Lastly apply a tonic or astringent lotion to enhance the effect.

Oatmeal Mask
For any skin type.

2 tablespoons steel-cut oats
150 ml (¼ pint) water
Boil oats and water gently about five minutes and strain off the liquid.

Apply liquid to the face and neck, leaving to dry on as long as necessary — several hours if you wish.

This is a gentle face-lift for a sagging face after illness or depression.

Rinse off, then apply a moisturising lotion.

Chamomile and Honey Mask
A gentle face mask for sensitive skin.

2 tablespoons unprocessed bran
3 tablespoons standard chamomile flower
infusion (p. 39)
1 teaspoon melted honey
Mix all ingredients together.

This is crumbly, but smooth it over the face and neck and leave ten minutes. Wash off with a mild or diluted chamomile infusion and blot dry.

Comfrey Mask
For any skin type.

*4 tablespoons standard comfrey
leaf infusion (p. 39)
½ teaspoon arrowroot
2 teaspoons apricot oil*

Pour comfrey infusion into a glass jar and stand in hot water. Stir in the arrowroot and heat until the liquid clears and thickens slightly. Remove from the heat, add the oil and shake well. Leave to cool.

Apply to the face and neck and allow to dry on ten to fifteen minutes. Rinse off, then moisturise with a lotion.

Dandelion Mask
For oily skin.

*6 fresh dandelion leaves
½ cup unpasteurised cow's milk or goat's
milk
1 tablespoon buttermilk
oatmeal flour to thicken*

Tear up and bruise the dandelion leaves and simmer them gently in the milk for five minutes. Set aside to steep and cool.

Strain off the milk, add the buttermilk and thicken to a thin paste with oatmeal flour. Leave to stand about five minutes while the oatmeal swells and absorbs some of the moisture.

Spread over face and neck and leave to dry on ten to fifteen minutes.

Wash off with tepid water.

Violet, Comfrey and Dandelion Mask
For normal to oily skin.

1 tablespoon mild violet leaf infusion (p. 39)
1 tablespoon mild dandelion infusion (p. 39)
1 tablespoon comfrey root decoction (see below)
1 tablespoon yoghurt
kaolin powder to thicken

For the decoction, simmer half a tablespoon of comfrey root in one cup of water for half an hour. Steep until cold.

Combine the liquids and yoghurt and thicken with kaolin to a soft paste.

Apply to the face and leave about fifteen to twenty minutes until set. Wash off with tepid water.

Chamomile, Licorice and Fennel Mask
For normal to oily skin.

2 tablespoons fennel seed infusion (see below)
2 tablespoons mild chamomile infusion (p. 39)
1 teaspoon licorice root powder
1 tablespoon honey
oatmeal flour to thicken

To make fennel seed infusion, infuse half a tablespoon crushed fennel seed in half a cup of boiling water until cold.

Combine the infusions, the licorice powder and the honey, then thicken to a soft paste with the oatmeal flour. Remember that oatmeal will swell up and absorb more moisture when combined with liquids and left to stand for five minutes.

Apply to the face and neck and leave on fifteen to twenty minutes until set. Wash off with tepid water.

Lemongrass Mask
For normal to oily skin.

3 tablespoons mild lemongrass infusion (p. 39)
1 tablespoon buttermilk
1 teaspoon honey
oatmeal flour to thicken

Combine the lemongrass, buttermilk and honey, and thicken to a soft paste with the oatmeal. Leave to stand about five minutes for the oatmeal flour to swell. Should the mixture then appear too stiff, add a little extra lemongrass infusion.

Apply to the face and neck, leaving fifteen to twenty minutes to set. Wash off with tepid water.

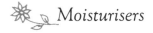 *Moisturisers*

Marshmallow and Comfrey Lotion
For normal to dry skin.

4 teaspoons marshmallow root decoction (see below)
2 teaspoons comfrey root decoction (see below)
1 teaspoon apricot oil
¼ teaspoon rosewater (from chemist) or
1 teaspoon rose infusion (see below)

Simmer one level tablespoon of dried marshmallow root in one cup water for half an hour to make a decoction. Leave to cool, then strain. Use half a level tablespoon of dried comfrey root to one cup water to make the comfrey root decoction, and proceed as for the marshmallow root decoction.

To make rose infusion, soak the petals of one rose in half a cup of boiling water, steeping for several hours.

Combine the ingredients and shake well.

'Milk of Roses'

①

1 oz	Almond Oil
1 oz	Spermaceti
½ pint	Rosewater
5 drops	tincture of Benzoin

Melt the wax, mix and warm rosewater
and benzoin, and add drop by drop
to the oils beating all the time.

②

4 drachms	tincture of Benzoin
1 oz	Glycerine
1 oz	Spermaceti
2 oz	Almond oil
½ pint	Rosewater

Mix rosewater, benzoin, and glycerine
and set on the hob to get lukewarm.
In the meantime put the almond
oil and spermaceti in a basin on the
fire in a pan of boiling water.
When melted add the rosewater, etc.
stirring and beating the whole time.
When mixed remove from the fire
and allow to cool. This is perhaps
the better recipe of the two.

'How to be Beautiful' 1913

Bran and Fennel Lotion
For normal to oily skin.

12 tablespoons bran water (see below)
3 tablespoons fennel infusion (see below)
To make bran water, follow the instructions given in the recipe for Houseleek, Rose and Comfrey Lotion, p. 63.

For fennel infusion, infuse two teaspoons of crushed fennel seed in half a cup of boiling water until cold and strain.

Combine the ingredients in a small glass bottle, screw on the lid and shake.

Floral Lotion
A light refining lotion for normal skin.

½ teaspoon lavender infusion
½ teaspoon chamomile infusion
½ teaspoon elderflower infusion
2 teaspoons almond oil
2 drops rosewater (from the chemist)
Make weak herbal infusions (p. 39). (Steep the lavender until cold.) Put all the ingredients in a small glass jar with a lid and shake well.

Lavender Lotion
A very light moisturiser
for normal skin.

1 tablespoon weak lavender infusion (p. 39)
1 teaspoon apricot oil
1 teaspoon Irish moss gel (p. 39)
Steep lavender until cold.

Combine the ingredients in a glass jar with a lid, and shake well.

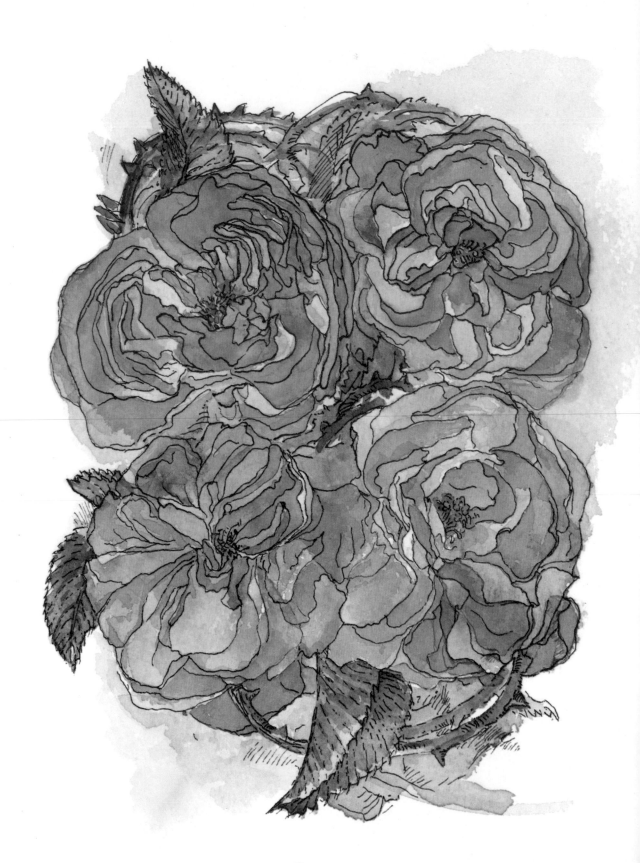

Roses

Violet Complexion Milk
Softening and refining to any skin type.

24 violet flowers
150 ml (¼ pint) distilled water
2 tablespoons almond meal

Put the almond meal and water in the blender for two minutes, or place in a screw-top jar and shake until milky. Pour into a non-metal pan, add the violet flowers and gently heat. Do not bring to the boil. Allow to cool, then strain and bottle.

Houseleek, Rose and Comfrey Lotion
For any skin type.

1 teaspoon houseleek juice (see below)
1 teaspoon rose infusion (see below)
2 teaspoons comfrey root decoction (see below)
1 teaspoon bran water (see below)
1 tablespoon quince gel (p. 41)

Houseleek juice is pressed from the fresh leaf.

To make the rose infusion, soak the petals of one rose in half a cup of boiling water, steeping until cold.

Simmer half a level tablespoon of dried comfrey root in one cup of water for half an hour to make a decoction.

To make bran water, bring gently to the boil one tablespoon of bran and one cup of water. Simmer three minutes, then allow to stand and cool. Strain the water off through cheesecloth, into a jar. Discard the bran.

Combine the ingredients in a small glass jar, screw on the lid and shake well.

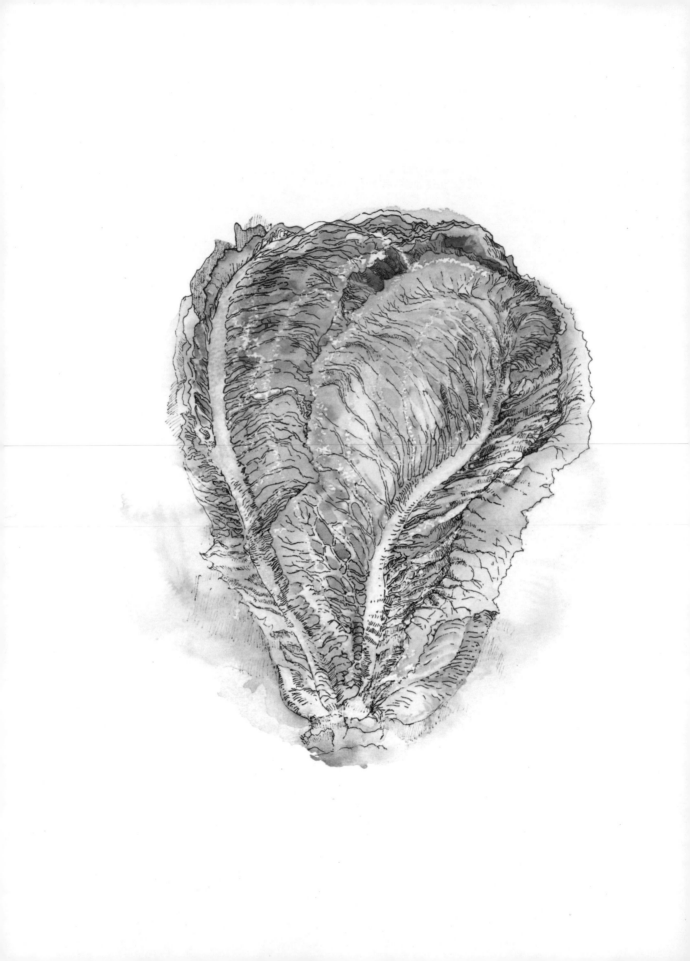

Lettuce Lotion
For normal skin.

1 teaspoon fresh lettuce juice (see below)
1 teaspoon liquid lecithin
½ teaspoon almond oil
½ teaspoon arrowroot gel (p. 40)

Put a fresh lettuce leaf through the juice extractor to obtain the lettuce juice. You may prefer to dilute it by taking half a teaspoon of juice and mixing it with half a teaspoon of distilled water.

Combine ingredients in a small glass jar; screw on the lid and shake well.

Almond and Apricot Lotion
For dry skin.

2 teaspoons almond milk
1 teaspoon apricot oil
⅓ teaspoon pumpkin seed oil

Combine ingredients and shake well.

Houseleek Lotion
For normal skin.

1 teaspoon liquid lecithin
1 teaspoon houseleek juice (see below)
½ teaspoon almond oil
1 teaspoon quince gel (p. 41)

Place one teaspoon of lecithin in a small glass jar. Take a fresh, succulent leaf of the houseleek plant and press it firmly to squeeze out one teaspoon of its natural juice. Add to the lecithin, then add remaining ingredients and shake.

Orange Flower Lotion
For any skin type.

*1 tablespoon orange flower toilet
water (p. 113)*
1 tablespoon quince gel (p. 41)
1 teaspoon almond oil (for normal skin)

For oily skin omit the oil; for dry skin use two teaspoons of oil. Combine the ingredients in a bottle, screw lid tightly and shake well. Rose toilet water (p. 113) makes a lovely substitute for the orange blossom in this lotion.

Chamomile and Fennel Lotion
For dry skin.

1 teaspoon fennel infusion (see below)
1 rounded teaspoon unsalted butter
2 teaspoons apricot oil
1 teaspoon mild chamomile infusion (p. 39)
1-2 drops lemon juice

Fennel infusion is made by adding one tablespoon crushed seeds to one cup boiling water, then allowing them to infuse until cold.

Melt the butter, add the oil, then the herbal infusions. Add the lemon juice. Stir or shake well. Use when slightly warm.

Lemongrass Lotion
For any skin type.

1 teaspoon apricot oil
½ teaspoon honey
2 teaspoons mild lemongrass infusion (p. 39)
1 drop cider vinegar

Combine the ingredients in a small glass bottle, screw the lid on firmly and shake.

freckles

$\frac{1}{4}$ pint Elderflower Water

$\frac{1}{4}$ pint thick Barley Water

$\frac{1}{2}$ pint spirits of Wine

Wash face frequently with this lotion and you will notice your freckles gradually disappear.

Fennel, Comfrey and Wych Hazel Lotion
For dry skin.

1 teaspoon fennel infusion (see below)
½ teaspoon comfrey root decoction (see below)
2 teaspoons unsalted butter
2 capsules wheatgerm oil
½ teaspoon distilled wych hazel (from chemist)

To make fennel infusion, infuse one tablespoon of crushed fennel seed in one cup of boiling water until cold.

To make comfrey root decoction, simmer half a tablespoon of dried comfrey root in one cup of water for half an hour. Steep until cold.

Melt the butter, add the oil, the wych hazel and the herb liquids. Stir well.

Use lotion while slightly warm.

Wych Hazel and Rose Lotion
For any skin type.

1 teaspoon almond oil
1 teaspoon rosewater or infusion (p. 39)
1½ teaspoons distilled wych hazel (from
chemist)
1 teaspoon honey
Combine the ingredients in a small glass bottle. Warm slightly if the honey needs softening. Screw on lid and shake well.

Fennel Lotion
A softening and healing lotion for dry skin.

1 teaspoon fennel infusion (see below)
1 tablespoon quince gel (p. 41)
1 teaspoon apricot oil
⅓ teaspoon pumpkin oil
To make fennel infusion, pour one cup boiling water over one tablespoon crushed seed and steep until cold.

Combine ingredients in a small glass jar and shake well.

Elderflower and Cucumber Lotion
For any skin type.

2 teaspoons mild elderflower infusion (p. 39)
1 teaspoon cucumber juice
1 teaspoon almond oil
2 tablespoons almond milk
1 drop tincture of benzoin
Combine the ingredients in a small glass jar, screw on the lid and shake vigorously.

Lavender, Rose and Comfrey Lotion
For normal skin.

2 teaspoons oatmeal water (see below)
2 tablespoons quince gel (p. 41)
2-4 teaspoons apricot oil
1 teaspoon lavender infusion (see below)
1 teaspoon rosehip decoction (see below)
1 teaspoon comfrey root decoction (p. 40)

Boil two tablespoons of steel-cut oats in one small cup of water for five minutes for oatmeal water, and strain. For lavender infusion, soak one teaspoon dried lavender in one cup of boiling water until cold. Simmer twelve fresh rosehips in one cup of water for half an hour for the rose decoction. For the comfrey root decoction, simmer half a tablespoon of dried comfrey root in one cup of water for half an hour, and steep until cold.

Combine the ingredients in a glass jar, screw on the lid and shake well.

Honey and Almond Face Softener
For any skin type. Nice for the hands,
too.

Melt together equal quantities of honey, white beeswax and almond oil. Pour into a small glass jar and screw on the lid. Shake vigorously.

Apply generously to face and neck, smoothing over without dragging the skin. Use warm.

Leave on fifteen to twenty minutes, then wash off with tepid water. Leaves the skin soft and supple.

Use occasionally.

Buttermilk and Marigold Lotion
A lovely day or night lotion which
balances the skin's acid mantle.

2 teaspoons buttermilk
2 teaspoons apricot oil
½ teaspoon almond oil
1 teaspoon standard marigold (or cowslip)
infusion (p. 39)

Steep the marigold infusion until cold —
no need to strain.

Combine ingredients in a small glass jar
with a lid and shake well.

Elderflower and Buttermilk Lotion
For normal to dry skin.

4 teaspoons buttermilk
2 teaspoons mild elderflower infusion (p. 39)
1 teaspoon apricot oil
2 teaspoons almond oil

Place the ingredients in a glass jar, screw
the lid on firmly and shake well.

Orange Flower Cream
For dry skin.

4 tablespoons orange flower toilet
water (p. 113)
1 teaspoon beeswax
¼ teaspoon honey
4 tablespoons almond oil

Put the beeswax, almond oil and honey
in a jar standing in hot water and stir
until they are melted. Continue stirring
vigorously while pouring in the orange
flower water. Remove the jar from the
hot water, then stir again until cool.
Apply sparingly to the face and neck.

Chian Earth

But of ye Chian, that
which is white, & drawing to
an ashy colour & that which is
like to ye Samian is to be taken:
but it is crusty, & white, but differing
in ye forms of ye making up. But it hath ye
same virtue that ye Samian hath. And it
makes ye visage, and more ye whole body to be
without wrinkles and clear, & in a bath it
scours instead of Nitre.

Dioscorides

A.D. 60

Gosmore

(Hypochaeris Maculata)

This plant is very useful to the
ladies, and ought to be found
upon their toilets. Its decoction
will take away freckles which are
brought on by the heat of the sun.
It is so innocent, that no harm need
be feared from its application.

Culpeper 1653

Licorice Cream
For dry skin.

1 teaspoon cocoa butter
1 teaspoon anhydrous lanolin (wool fat)
1 tablespoon apricot oil
1 teaspoon standard comfrey leaf
infusion (p. 39)
1 teaspoon standard chamomile flower
infusion (p. 39)
¼ teaspoon licorice root powder

Melt the cocoa butter and lanolin in a jar
standing in hot water. Add the oil and
stir in. Add the herbal infusions and the
licorice powder. Remove from hot water,
screw the lid firmly on the jar and shake
until cool.

Rose, Honey and Almond Cream
For dry skin.

1 teaspoon standard rose petal infusion (see
below)
½ teaspoon beeswax
2 teaspoons cocoa butter
2 teaspoons almond oil
2 teaspoons apricot oil
¼ teaspoon honey

To make rose infusion, soak the petals of
one rose in half a cup of boiling water,
steeping for several hours.

Melt beeswax in a glass jar standing in
hot water, then add cocoa butter and
wait for it to melt. Pour in the oils, then
the honey and make sure it is all melted.
Add the rose petal infusion. Remove the
jar from the hot water, screw on the cap
and shake until cool.

To Makeup or Not to Makeup

Healthy, beautiful skin needs no adornment or concealment. The use of makeup is, of course, a very personal choice. It's up to you. However, remember that when you use makeup you put most of the time and effort into getting the makeup looking right. When you don't use makeup, all your effort goes into getting your skin looking right. To me, that is the essence of beauty.

Have you ever stopped to consider why you use makeup? After all, it is not a necessity, but a convention. Towards the end of the nineteenth century, when women began rebelling against repression, the use of makeup by those other than actresses was regarded as a break-through to freedom, for in Queen Victoria's day, makeup was considered immoral. Nice girls didn't use it.

As makeup became popular, lucrative business enterprises were set up, accompanied by lavish advertising to influence feminine appearance. Women looking for a style upon which to model themselves tried to copy the faces of their favourite film stars. It was a morale booster. Fashion followed fashion.

Now, a century later, women are becoming more individual, more secure in being who they are. The conforming mask of makeup is no longer a necessity; it is a personal decision. Women feel free to please themselves.

I consider makeup detrimental because powder and powder-base are drying to the skin and clogging to the pores, restricting natural respiratory and eliminatory functions. A matt look is aging, while a glossy look is artificial.

If you are unused to going without it, you will feel naked and unadorned without makeup at first; your skin may not look very attractive. It may be a bad colour, over-shiny, veined, pored, in fact revealing all the problems you have been so carefully concealing under your powder and paint, instead of dealing with directly.

If your diet is wholesome and balanced and you are not subjected to undue stress, then your skin will very quickly respond to freedom from cosmetics. However, it needs just as much time and care and love as before to keep it beautiful. It will still get dirty every day from pollution in the air, it will dehydrate in dry conditions of summer or winter, so its moisture content will be depleted. It will need toning and softening and protecting from the elements. You will still need to follow a regular skin-care routine.

The colour of your skin will improve once it is given the chance to breathe and return to its own natural balance with the use of simple lotions and herbal infusions. The skin's texture will improve because the function of herbal preparations is to balance the skin, not conceal it.

Admittedly, the first two or three weeks without makeup can take a certain amount of courage, because there are moments when you know you look dreadful. Don't run back to the makeup jar. Be patient. Try various herbal infusions, cleansers, toners, lotions, and establish a routine which suits your skin. It is worth the effort!

Specific Skin Problems

Lines and Wrinkles

Lines and wrinkles on the face come about through loss of skin tone because elasticity lessens, as does the skin's ability to hold moisture. The skin has a protective acid mantle which is made alkaline by such things as soap, water and makeup. Restoring the normal acid-alkali balance is an important step towards restoring and maintaining skin tone.

Certain areas of the skin most subject to over-use become affected first. These are the forehead, around the eyes, around the mouth, and the neck. With the exception of the skin under the eyes, these special areas can be gently worked on morning and night, with cleansers, toners and moisturisers. Lines and wrinkles are encouraged by such factors as poor diet, insufficient sleep, bad posture when in bed, stresses and tensions, overwork, eyestrain, pollution, air-conditioning and central heating.

Spots and Blemishes

Keep your skin clean by using a non-oily bran or oatmeal cleanser (pp. 42, 44). Restore the acid balance by rinsing with one teaspoon of cider vinegar diluted with two tablespoons of distilled water.

Compresses for Disturbed Skin   Compresses, which enable a generous quantity of herbal infusion to be applied and held to the skin, are valuable in helping to clear up spots and blemishes. To make a compress, dip sterile gauze or cottonwool into a warm infusion of the herb and hold it against the skin for fifteen minutes. If the fresh bruised herb is being used, press it on to the affected skin, or place it inside some cheesecloth if preferred.

To apply a compress to the entire facial area, cut out a cottonwool mask with two holes for the eyes and another for the mouth and nostril area. Moisten the cottonwool in the infusion and apply to the face while lying down.

Use any of the following cleansing and healing herbs as a compress:

Comfrey Compress

Make a decoction by simmering 15 g (½ oz) of the chopped, dried comfrey root or 30 g (1 oz) of the scrubbed, sliced fresh root, in 500 ml (1 pint) water for half an hour. Allow to cool until comfortably warm before using. The allantoin contained in the root is the regenerative and healing agent.

Chamomile Compress

Make a weak infusion (p. 39) of the dried flowers. Strain and allow to cool until reasonably warm before using. Chamomile is cleansing and strengthening to the skin, reducing any puffiness of the tissues.

Coltsfoot Compress

Infuse one teaspoon of the dried leaves in one cup of boiling water for ten minutes. Strain and allow to cool before using. Coltsfoot is an emollient and anti-inflammatory herb.

Cowslip Compress

Make an infusion by pouring one cup of boiling water over one and a half teaspoons of dried flowers. Infuse five minutes, then strain and cool sufficiently for use. Cowslip is cleansing and soothing.

Cleavers Compress

Take six fresh, 5 cm (2 in) sprigs of leaves, and pour one cup of boiling water over them. Allow them to infuse until the water is cool enough to use. Cleavers is a cleansing herb.

Burdock Compress

Place one tablespoon of chopped dried burdock root in one cup of cold water. Heat gently and simmer for five minutes. Strain before use. Burdock is cleansing and healing, useful for skin irritations.

Pansy Compress

Soak two to four teaspoons of the whole herb in one cup of water for an hour. Then gently heat and simmer twenty seconds. Remove from the heat, infuse ten minutes. Strain and cool before use. Pansy is a cooling, emollient and anti-inflammatory herb.

Dandelion Compress

Take three teaspoons of chopped fresh leaves and cover them with a small cup of cold water. Gently heat and simmer five minutes. Strain and cool before use. Dandelion is a cleansing herb.

Violet Compress

This herb is best used fresh. The leaves and flowers of violet contain a high proportion of vitamins A and C, as well as salicylic acid, making it a very cleansing and healing herb. Bruise the leaves or flowers and apply them to the face.

Chickweed Compress

Chickweed is best used fresh. Pick the leaves, bruise them and apply them to the face. A cleansing and healing herb capable of drawing impurities out of the skin.

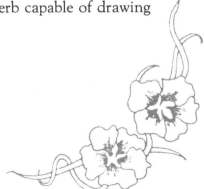

Remedy Against a Mole

Berries - of - the - h'as - plant
mamer - grain
Pound, and let the person take
who has the mole.

Honey
Leaf - of - the - mamer - corn.
Crush in Water - with - which - the
Phallus - has - been - washed: therewith
plaster it one night that it may remain
on his arms and his limbs.

'The Papyrus Ebers' 1500 B.C.

Marigold Wash

An infusion of marigold flowers is suitable for washing blemishes, particularly on an oily skin. Combine it with more emollient herbs such as chamomile and comfrey for a dry skin.

To make a marigold infusion, take the petals of two flowers, pour over half a cup of boiling water and infuse until cold.

Marigold flowers may be steeped in cider vinegar in a screw-top jar for a week. Then strain off and bottle the vinegar. To make a facial wash which heals as well as restoring the acid mantle to the skin, dilute one teaspoon of vinegar with two tablespoons of water. Fresh new leaves may be substituted for flowers when the latter are not available.

Combine three tablespoons of standard marigold infusion (p. 39) with one tablespoon of distilled wych hazel (from the chemist) to make an astringent and healing lotion.

Lemon Balm Wash

A mild infusion (p. 39) is helpful for oily skin which needs a gentle cleansing to help clear up pimples.

Houseleek Lotion

Take a fresh, succulent leaf from the houseleek plant and press it firmly to squeeze out the juice. The clear liquid is anti-inflammatory and mildly astringent, two properties which are helpful in clearing blemished skin.

Violet Lotion

Make a lotion by putting a handful of fresh violet leaves through the juice extractor. Use the green liquid to soothe and heal spots and blemishes.

Licorice Powder

The brown-coloured powdered root of the licorice plant may be applied to spots to help them to dry and heal.

Cinquefoil Wash

Make a mild infusion by pouring one cup of boiling water over three level tablespoons of fresh, chopped cinquefoil leaves. Steep one hour. Use as an astringent wash for oily, blemished skin.

Quick Remedies for Occasional Pimples

Marigold

Take a petal of the orange-coloured calendula marigold, bruise it gently between the fingers and press on to the spot. Hold it there about two minutes. Repeat from time to time, but don't fuss over it. This simple application will heal a pimple overnight, leaving just a trace of redness. Another petal pressed on in the morning will remove the redness completely in a few hours. The healing action takes place almost miraculously while you are getting on with your life. This remedy will also flatten out white lumps under the skin.
If a flower is not available, use a calendula leaf in the same way.

Castor Oil

Castor oil has very powerful drawing properties, so if you get one of those large, boil-like pimples, bring it to a head by applying a dab of castor oil night and morning.

Honey

Honey is an alternative for dealing with a large, angry pimple. Apply a dab night and morning to draw it up to a head.

Age Spots
or Brown Pigmentation

Rub castor oil into the skin night and morning to remove the freckle-like brown patches (liver marks) which appear on mature skin. Other oils to try are St John's wort and eucalyptus.

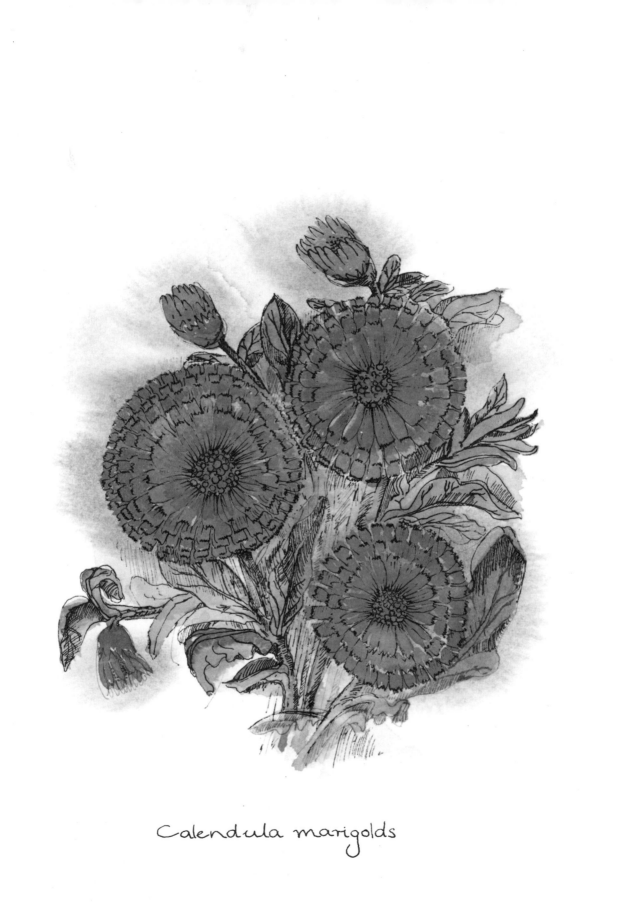

Calendula marigolds

Shiny Noses

This is a very common trouble.
When it is present wash the
face first with hot and then cold
water, and always use your oatmeal
bag. After doing so apply this lotion
to the nose, leaving it to dry on.

2oz   Rosewater
1oz   Eau de Cologne

Mix and shake well.

'Madame Cristo's Beauty Guide'

1923

Cresses (Water)
(Sisymbrium Nasturtium
Aquatica)

The leaves bruised, or the juice,
is good to be applied to the face
or other parts troubled with freckles,
pimples, spots, or the like, at night,
and washed away in the morning.

Culpeper 1653

Fumitory (Fumaria Officinalis)

The juice of the Fumitory and docks
mingled with vinegar, and the places
gently washed or wet therewith, cures
all sorts of scabs, pimples, blotches,
wheals, and pushes which rise on
the face or hands, or any other
parts of the body.

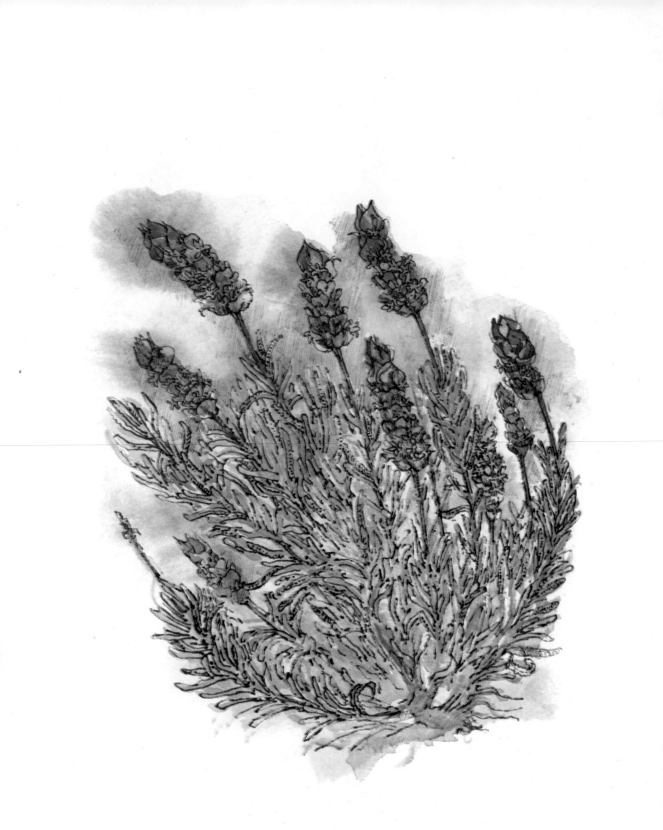

Lavender

❀ Blackheads

For skin afflicted with blackheads, cleanse thoroughly with almond meal or oatmeal mixed with some buttermilk. Candied honey, slightly thinned with water, is effective too.

After cleansing, apply a compress using a standard infusion of dandelion, parsley, yarrow or lemongrass (p. 39).

Ensure the acid balance of the skin is correct by rinsing occasionally with one teaspoon of apple cider vinegar diluted in two tablespoons of distilled water.

Never pick or squeeze out blackheads with the fingernails. Use two cotton buds to press the skin around them, making them pop out. Be gentle, don't use force.

❀ Large Pores

Large pores are usually associated with oily skin. To improve the appearance of the skin, cleanse with almond meal or oatmeal, then apply a fifteen-minute compress of a mild infusion of horsetail, marigold petals or sage leaves (p. 39).

At other times use refining lotions such as buttermilk, or comfrey root, lavender or parsley infusions (p. 39).

Large pores may also appear in dry skin where creams or heavy oils have been used. Avoid creams wherever possible and use lotions which are light and refining to the skin.

To reduce the size of the pores use a mild freshener, toner or mask (see recipe section p. 50).

❀ Thread Veins

Thread veins are the small, red, broken veins showing in the skin and giving it a somewhat weatherbeaten look.

If your skin is troubled by this condition, don't expose it to extremes of temperature, and avoid tea, coffee and alcohol which tend to cause dilation of facial veins. Eat lots of foods containing vitamin C, like rosehip, citrus juice and peel, parsley, violet leaves and capsicum (green pepper).

The traditional herb for improving thread veins is coltsfoot, applied as a tepid compress. Add a teaspoon of dried leaves to 150 ml (¼ pint) boiling water, infuse ten minutes, then strain.

If the skin is very dry, rub over a small amount of almond oil before applying the compress.

THE EYES

The skin under the eye is very thin and delicate. Leave it alone at night, then if any puffiness should occur around the eyes, the skin is more likely to retain its elasticity and not become unduly stretched.

A variety of herbs and plants are effective in reducing puffiness and toning the skin.

If you are in a hurry in the morning cut a slice of cucumber and rub this over the eyelid and the skin below the eye. Keep your eyes closed for two to three minutes to allow the juice to dry. Later, pat on, do not rub, a minute drop of light oil such as vitamin E or apricot.

If you haven't a cucumber handy, cut a slice of raw potato and gently rub it over the eye area in the same way. After about fifteen minutes, splash with cold water, pat dry with a tissue, then apply a minute dab of light oil.

If you have time to lie down for ten to fifteen minutes, moisten two pads of cottonwool with a little distilled wych hazel (from the chemist) and place over each eye. Don't have the cottonwool so wet that the liquid runs into your eyes.

Herbs suitable for making infusions and compresses to reduce puffiness around the eyes are: comfrey leaf, parsley, rosehip, lemon verbena leaves, chamomile flowers, coltsfoot leaves.

All of these should be used only when freshly made as weak infusions (p. 39) allowed to cool to a tepid temperature. Don't put anything stale near your eyes. Use fresh, clean cottonwool or sterile lint for bathing or making compresses.

Herbs suitable for making compresses or infusions to bathe tired eyes are: parsley, fennel seed, chamomile flowers, cornflowers, coltsfoot leaves, borage leaves, white rose petals and elderflowers.

As far as wrinkles and fine lines under the eyes are concerned, the golden rule is don't overdo any treatment to this area, or you'll make more wrinkles. Keep all the toners, masks and fresheners you use on your face well away from this area. Don't apply creams or heavy oil as they stretch the skin. Be very sparing with lotions or light oils.

To tone occasionally, use freshly made almond milk (p. 54) gently patted on.

The juice of the houseleek is also soothing and mildly astringent for use on the delicate skin under the eyes. The houseleek is *not* the ordinary onion-flavoured garden leek, but a totally different plant. It is a succulent with thick greyish-green leaves, and it is the juice pressed out of the leaves that is used. For a more detailed description of the houseleek, see p. 181.

As a special treatment when the lines under the eyes have become very hard, apply houseleek juice in the morning and leave to dry on. Two or three hours later, slightly warm half a teaspoon of honey and mix in with it two drops (a quarter of a teaspoon) of almond oil. Carefully slide on to the area a large, generous dab of this prepared honey. Lie down fifteen minutes, so that you will not drag the skin. Wash off with pads of cottonwool, generously soaked in a tepid chamomile infusion (p. 39), so that the liquid melts away the honey without pulling the skin. Do this for two or three days in succession.

Remedy for the Eye
When Something Evil
Has Happened to It.

A Human Brain
Divide it in halves

To one half add Honey and anoint the Eye therewith in the Evening.

Dry the other half, crush, powder, and anoint the Eye therewith in the Morning.

ANOTHER
to Drive Out Hotness
in the Eyes

Tallow - from - the - Jawbone -
of - an - Ass
Mix in Cool Water and let the
Patient put on his Temples in
order that he may be healed
forth with.

'The Papyrus Ebers'
1500 B.C.

Buttermilk tones under the eyes, restoring the acid balance to the skin. Leave to dry on.

Buttermilk toner, made according to the recipe on page 53, is beneficial too, softening hard lines and toning the skin.

The area above the eye, from the lid to the brow, should be treated in the same way as the under eye. It is delicate too, and can become stretched. If the skin of the eyelid is loose and flabby, gently but firmly press it back into place with the fingertips, several times a day.

Crowsfeet at the sides of the eyes will need constant attention. They will require lots of toning to tighten the skin, which has become tired and lost its resilience. Any of the facial toners (pp. 53-5) are suitable for this purpose.

THE NECK

Stimulate extra dry or wrinkled areas of the neck and under the chin where tone and elasticity have declined.

Apply an oatmeal mask made with steel-cut oats (p. 56). Leave on half an hour. Rinse off with a weak tepid infusion (p. 39) of one of the stimulating or tonic herbs, such as sage, thyme, peppermint, nettle, horsetail or limeflower. Pat dry and leave ten minutes before applying a moisturising lotion.

For daily use make a toning lotion of four tablespoons of mild elderflower infusion (p. 39) to one teaspoon of benzoin.

Thyme and Sage Neck Cream

1 teaspoon anhydrous lanolin (wool fat)
2 teaspoons apricot oil
2 teaspoons standard thyme infusion (p. 40)
2 teaspoons standard sage infusion (p. 40)

Melt the lanolin in a jar standing in hot water. Add the oil, then the herbal infusions. Remove jar from the water, screw on the cap and shake well.

Apply the cream to the neck, rubbing in thoroughly. Leave twenty minutes, then blot off the excess.

THE LIPS

The lips need softening and protecting just as regularly as the rest of the face. If they peel excessively, or are dry, lined or chapped, check your intake of vitamin B foods. Some of the sources are oatmeal, wheatgerm, bran, yeast, organ meats, free range eggs, yoghurt, goat's milk and sprouted seeds.

Pumpkin Oil Lip Softener

1 teaspoon coconut oil
½ teaspoon cocoa butter
½ teaspoon pumpkin oil

Melt all the ingredients together in a shallow glass container or small glass jar standing in a saucepan of hot water. Stir thoroughly or shake well, then leave to cool and set. Alternatively, pour into a discarded lipstick container and leave to cool and set.

Honey Lip Salve
Healing and soothing to dry or chapped lips.

1 tablespoon honey
½-1 teaspoon melted beeswax
2 teaspoons almond oil

Melt together the honey and beeswax. Add the almond oil. Put in a small screw top jar, and shake vigorously to emulsify.

Herbal Lip Cream

1 teaspoon anhydrous lanolin (wool fat)
1 teaspoon apricot oil
2 teaspoons standard marigold or chickweed
infusion (p. 39), or marshmallow root
decoction (see below)

To make marshmallow root decoction, simmer one level tablespoon of dried marshmallow root in one cup of water for half an hour. Leave to cool, then strain. Place the lanolin in a small glass jar in a hot water bath to melt. Add the oil and then the herb infusion or decoction. Remove jar from water bath, screw on cap and shake well. Leave to cool.

Peppermint Lip Salve

½ teaspoon beeswax
1 tablespoon cocoa butter
½-1 drop peppermint oil

Melt the beeswax in a small glass jar placed in hot water. Then add the cocoa butter, melting all together. To make half a drop of peppermint oil, put one drop of peppermint oil on a teaspoon with a dropper then tip the spoon and let the oil run off into the wax. If you prefer a stronger mentholation use one whole drop of peppermint oil. Remove jar from water bath, screw on cap and shake. Pour the liquid mixture into a discarded lipstick container and allow to cool and set.

THE TEETH

Fresh sage leaves rubbed over the teeth clean and polish them so they feel like silk. This is an old and tried method.

Another idea is to mash up a ripe strawberry and dip your toothbrush in it to clean your teeth. Rinse thoroughly afterwards. Use occasionally.

For a quick toothpowder, use orris root, if you are not averse to a slightly bitter taste.

Mouth Washes and Breath Fresheners

Should you wish to freshen your mouth, or sweeten your breath, try a standard infusion (p. 39) of one of the following herbs as a mouth wash: peppermint, spearmint, eau-de-cologne mint, lavender, cornflower, rosemary, sage, marjoram, pennyroyal, lemon balm, thyme, summer savory.

Alternatively, chew a sprig of parsley or a dried clove.

A drop of any herbal oil in half a glass of water makes a flavoured rinse.

To cleanse or heal the mouth and the tongue, make a mild infusion (p. 39) of violet flowers steeped half an hour, to use as a rinse. Hold the liquid in the mouth several minutes.

Herbal Toothpowder

1 tablespoon dried rosemary
1 teaspoon dried sage
1 tablespoon arrowroot
1 teaspoon orris root powder
½ teaspoon licorice root powder

Grind the dried rosemary leaves to a fine powder in a mortar and pestle. Gently shake through a fine sieve to remove any fibres. Follow the same procedure with the dried sage leaves. Combine all the ingredients in a small glass bottle and shake.

To use, put a small amount into the palm of the hand, and dip a wet toothbrush into the toothpowder.

Rinse your toothbrush thoroughly after use.

Simple Toothpaste

1 tablespoon powdered orris root
½ tablespoon quince gel (p. 41)
1 teaspoon diluted oil of peppermint or other
flavouring

Peppermint oil is very potent, so dilute it by adding one drop to 1 teaspoon of a bland vegetable oil such as sunflower, safflower or corn.

Other flavours you may prefer are clove, thyme, rosemary, anise, eucalyptus.

Mix the ingredients to a putty-like consistency. Store in a cool place in an airtight jar.

PART IV

THE BODY:
Bathing
Body Oils & Lotions
Deodorants
The Hands
The Feet
Care of the Body Outdoors
Exercise
A Healthy Diet

BATHING

As the skin is the only major organ we can see and touch it is amazing that we are not all more generally aware of the importance of skin functions. Skin is not merely a fancy wrapper — it is the largest organ of the body and is designed to excrete 30 per cent of the waste products. Your whole body should be looked after (not just your face) to promote healthy skin and general well-being.

Dry Bathing

For this you will need a sauna brush with a handle, or a loofah. Dry bathing consists of brushing all parts of the body below the neck, excluding (for women) delicate breast areas. Go very gently and lightly on the paler softer areas of the stomach and on the insides of the arms and legs. Brush for five to ten minutes every morning on rising, to stimulate the circulation and to rid the skin of accumulated dead cells, debris and toxins.

After brushing, apply a coating of light oil, such as apricot oil, all over the body. Leave for ten minutes, then towel off the excess, giving a vigorous rub.

Water Bathing

Brush the skin as in dry bathing, to improve the circulation and loosen dead skin cells. Rub over with diluted cider vinegar or scented herbal vinegar, the proportions being one part vinegar to eight parts distilled water, then rinse in a warm bath.

The cider vinegar will help to combat any dryness of the skin and restore the acid balance. It also invigorates the body.

Strip of its chaff and its coverings the barley which the Libyan husbandmen have sent in the ships. Let an equal quantity of vetches be made moist with ten eggs; but let the peeled barley amount to two pounds. When this has been dried in the airy breezes, bid the slow-moving ass bruise them with the rough mill-stone. Pound together also the first horns that fall from off the long-lived stag; of this make there to be the sixth part of a full pound. And when now they have been reduced to a fine powder, then sift them all in the hollow sieve. Add twice six bulbs of narcissus without the skin, which a strong right-hand must bruise in a clean mortar of marble; let it receive also two ounces of gum together with Etrurian spelt; to this let nine times as much more honey be contributed by you. Whoever shall rub her face with such a mixture, she will shine more brightly than her mirror.

Ovid   43 B.C. — A.D. 18

"De Medicamine faciei"

A Sweet-Scented Bath

Take of Roses, Citron peel,
sweet flowers, Orange flowers,
Jessamy, Bays, Rosemary,
Lavender, Mint, Pennyroyal, of each
a sufficient quantity, boil them
together gently and make a Bath to
which add Oyl of Spike six drops,
musk five grains, Ambergris three
grains.

The Receipt Book of John
Middleton 1734
Quoted in E.S. Rohde
'A Garden of Herbs'

Herbal Bathing

This is not a rinsing bath, but one in which to soak for at least twenty minutes. Get an inflatable plastic cushion on which to rest your head while you are lying soaking, and set an alarm clock so that you can relax without worrying how much time has elapsed. Don't go to sleep! Read if you wish or listen to some music on the radio.

Herbs for Bathing

Herbs used in baths are chosen according to the effect on the skin or body which one wishes to achieve (see below). Make a strong infusion (about 2 cups dried herb to 500 ml (1 pint) boiling water) of the herbs chosen, leave to steep until cool, strain and add to the bath water. Use herbs individually or in any combination that appeals.

To Sweetly Scent the Skin

Use any of the sweetly scented floral herbs or flowers like rose, violet, lavender, cowslip, meadowsweet, frangipani, sweet pea, orange flower, jasmine, honeysuckle, rose geranium, carnation.

Underline the perfumes by adding spicy herbs like lemon balm, rosemary, chamomile, eau-de-cologne mint, spearmint, clary sage, clove, lovage.

To Soften the Skin

Use emollient and cleansing herbs like chamomile, chickweed, cowslip, lettuce, marshmallow, marigold (with either comfrey or chamomile), pansy, violet leaf and flower, applemint, spearmint, elderflower, roses (flowers, leaves or hips), red clover, sage, comfrey, orange flowers, fennel seed.

To Remove Excess Oil from the Skin

Use astringent herbs that act on the sebaceous glands like clary sage, lemon verbena, red clover, lemongrass, comfrey, houseleek, wych hazel, lavender.

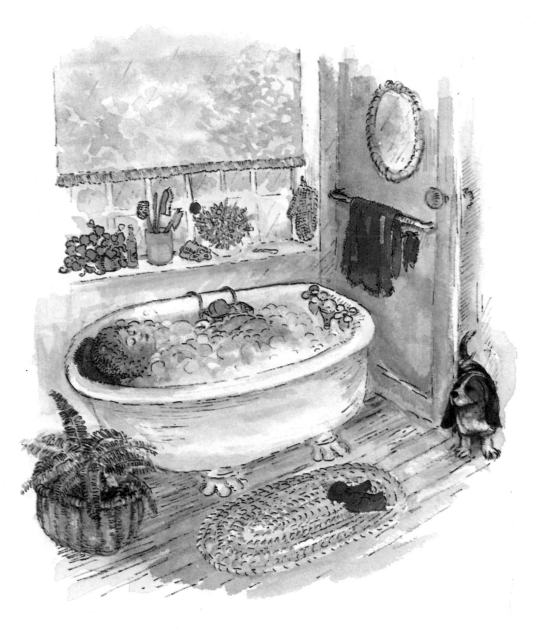

HYACINTH

The roots, after the opinion of
Dioscorides, being beaten and
applied with white Wine,
hinder or keepe back the
growth of haires.

Gerard's Harball

1597

Ninon de L'Enclos
Beauty Bath

Dissolve 8 ounces of kitchen salt
and 3½ ounces of carbonate
of soda in a quart of water.
 In 3 quarts of milk dissolve
3 pounds of honey.
Pour the first solution into the bath
and stir it well with the bath water.
Then pour in the second solution
 and stir again. The bath is
 then ready.

C.F. Leyel
'The Magic of Herbs'

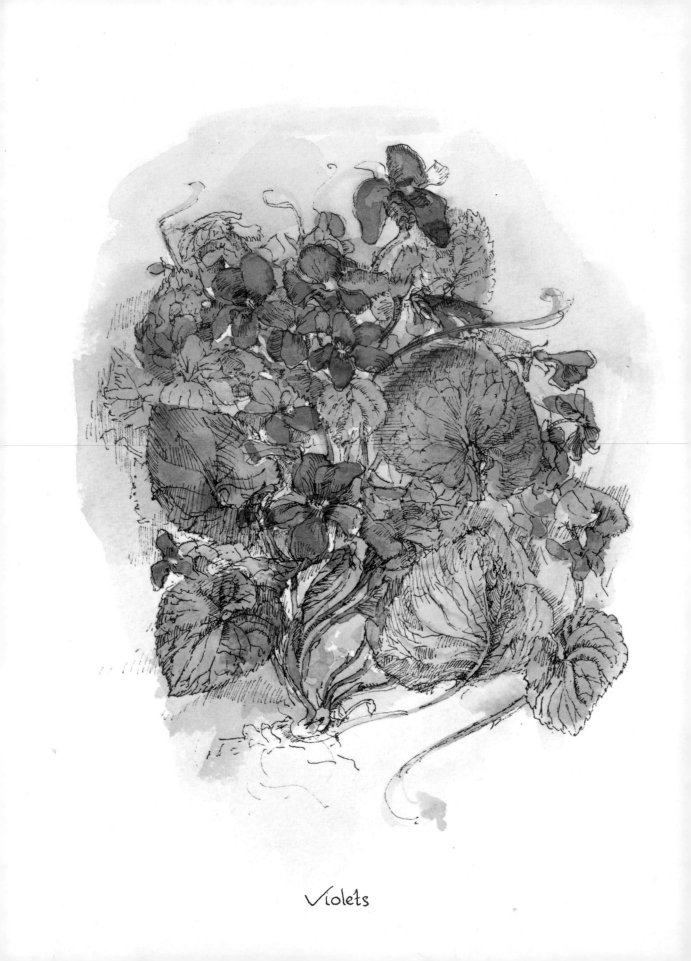

Violets

To Deodorise the Skin

Use herbs like lovage, cleavers or rosemary.

To Tone the Skin

Use tonic astringent and cleansing herbs like burdock root (with comfrey and fennel), cinquefoil, red clover, dandelion, peppermint, horsetail.

To Stimulate the Skin and the Body

Use stimulating and tonic herbs like rosemary, dandelion, hyssop (with mint and rosemary), lovage, marjoram, nettles, sage, savory, southernwood (with lemon balm or rosemary), thyme, comfrey.

Herbal Bath Bags

Take a piece of coarse cheesecloth, a handkerchief, or a thin towelling face cloth, and place two tablespoons of bran and one tablespoon of chamomile flowers on it. Gather up the ends and sides to make a bag and secure it with a twist, string or ribbon. Place the bag under the hot tap while the water is running into the bath. Before getting into the bath give the bag a few squeezes to release some of the milky bran and chamomile water. Use the bag to scrub yourself all over. Softening and pleasant.

Other Ingredients for Bath Bags

Three tablespoons of ground oatmeal to two tablespoons of powdered orris root for a delicate violet-scented bag, and two tablespoons of almond meal with a teaspoon of lavender flowers for a lavender perfume.

Using bran or oatmeal or almond meal as your basic scrubbing ingredient, combine with any of the aromatic herbs along with some chamomile or elderflowers to make your own choice of bath bag.

❋ Soap

The body may be kept adequately clean and refreshed without the use of soap. However, certain places where odours are more prevalent, under the arms and in the pubic area, do need a regular soaping. Always use a mild soap. Choose a soap free from colouring, synthetic perfumes, anti-oxidants and anti-bacterial ingredients. Pure soaps and castiles are available from the chemist if you do not wish to make your own at home.

It is possible to modify a cake of pure soap to make it into a herbal soap.

Herbal Soap

56 g (2 oz) pure soap
56 ml (2 oz) herbal infusion (p. 39)

Suitable herbs include comfrey, marshmallow, fennel, marigold and chamomile. Make a mild or standard infusion of the herb chosen, depending on the strength you prefer. Strain before use.

Place the herbal infusion in a jar standing in hot water. Grate the soap, then slowly add to the infusion, stirring in and melting it. Stir until the soap and the herb are thoroughly combined. Line a plastic soap dish with a damp cloth and press in the dough-like soap mixture to make a cake. Leave to set, dry and harden, for one or two days. Lift the cake of soap out of the dish with the cloth (which may then be discarded). Wrap in greaseproof paper.

Almond Meal Soap Substitute
A non-sudsing but very gentle and
softening soap substitute.

2 tablespoons almond meal
2 tablespoons kaolin powder (from the
chemist)
2 teaspoons almond oil
Mix together and mould into a knob.
Add a drop of any herbal oil to perfume
if desired. Lavender, rosemary or jasmine
would be nice.

What then is called the 'royal' unguent,
because it is a blend prepared for the
kings of Parthia, is made of behen-nut
juice, costus, amomum, Syrian cinnamon
cardomon, spikenard, cat-thyme,
myrrh, cinnamon-bark, styrax-tree,
gum, ladanum, balm, Syrian reed
and Syrian rush, wild grape, cinnamon
leaf, serichatum, cyprus, rosewood,
all-heal, saffron, gladiolus, marjoram,
lotus, honey and wine.

PLINY - the Elder
A.D. 23 - 79

'Natural History'

Eau de Cologne

One pint rectified spirits, one ounce orange flower water, two drams oil of bergamot, two drams oil of lemon, twenty minims oil of rosemary, twenty minims oil of neroli. Allow the mixture to stand for a couple of months, thoroughly shaking at intervals. Filter if necessary.

Mrs. Charles Roundell
'The Still Room'

Quoted by E.S. Rohde
'A Garden of Herbs'

BODY OILS & LOTIONS

Body Oils

Almond oil is my favourite because it is light and easily absorbed. It can be used alone or combined with a little cider vinegar or lemon juice when it is both softening and invigorating to the skin.

Olive oil, combined with coconut oil, and perfumed with a drop of rosemary oil, is good for massaging the body.

A few drops of pumpkin oil added to a tablespoon of apricot oil is soothing and healing to dry skin.

Herbal oils made from marigold or chamomile flowers are healing to the skin.

The sweet-scented yellow wallflower may be made into a herbal oil which is soothing to the nerves and the muscles.

The bright yellow flowers and the leaves of St John's wort make an oil soothing to the nerves and the body.

To make herbal oils crush a handful of the fresh herb with a mortar and pestle with the addition of a little white vinegar. Place the herb and vinegar in a jar, and pour in sufficient almond oil to just cover the herb. Screw on the lid tightly and shake the jar. Stand in a warm or sunny place for about three weeks, shaking every day. It may be necessary to strain off the oil and add fresh herbs, repeating the process, to obtain sufficient herbal strength.

Body Lotions

Elderflower Body Lotion

Make a mild infusion of elderflower (p. 39), adding half a teaspoon of tincture of benzoin to a cup of herb water if you want extra toning. Mildly stimulating to the skin.

Rosemary and Vinegar Body Lotion

Dilute one teaspoon of cider vinegar with two tablespoons of a mild rosemary decoction (p. 40) to make a refreshing body lotion.

Rosewater Body Lotion

Refer to the recipe for rose petal skin freshener on page 52 for a fragrant body lotion.

Wych Hazel and Herb Body Lotion

Make a fragrant, refreshing and toning body lotion by steeping herbs in an equal quantity of distilled wych hazel from the chemist. Place ingredients in an airtight jar at room temperature for two weeks.
Strain off the liquid and bottle.
Combinations of herbs:
1. Mint, rosemary, lavender leaves.
2. Lavender flowers, rosemary, peppermint, comfrey, lemon thyme, rose petals.
3. Peppermint, comfrey, sage, rosemary, lemon verbena.

Rose, Honey and Almond Body Lotion

1 tablespoon quince gel (p. 41)
1½ teaspoons almond oil
¼ teaspoon honey
1 teaspoon strong chamomile infusion (p. 39)
1 drop rosewater (from the chemist)
Combine ingredients in a small glass jar,
screw on the lid and shake well.

Hungary – Water : From Mrs. Du Pont, of Lyons; which is the same, Which has been famous about Montpelier. — Take to every gallon of Brandy, or clean Spirits, one handful of Rosemary, one handful of Lavender. I suppose the handfuls to be about a foot long a-piece; and these Herbs must be cut in Pieces about an Inch long. Put these to infuse in the Spirits, and with them, about one handful of Myrtle cut as before. When this has stood three Days, distil it, and you will have the finest Hungary-Water that can be....

R. Bradley 'The Country Housewife and Lady's Director 1732

Quoted in E.S. Rohde 'A Garden of Herbs'

Orange-Flower Water

Take four pounds of unpicked Orange Flowers, bruise them in a marble mortar, and pour on them nine quarts of clear water. Distil in a cold still and draw off five or six quarts, which will be exquisitely fragrant. If you are desirous of having it still higher flavoured, draw off at first seven quarts, unlute the still, and throw away the residue; empty back the water already distilled, and add to it two pounds of Orange Flowers bruised. Again luting the Still, repeat the distillation, and draw off five or six quarts. Then top, being careful not to draw off too much water, lest the Flowers should become dry and burn-to.

The Toilet of Flora
1776

Toilet Waters

Toilet waters to delicately perfume the skin may be made from freshly picked sweetly scented flowers and leaves.

Orange Flower Toilet Water

1½ large cups fresh orange blossom
700 ml (24 fl oz) boiling water
2 tablespoons gin or brandy

Pour the boiling water over the orange blossom. Cover and leave to infuse at room temperature twenty-four hours, then in the refrigerator for a further two days. Strain and add gin or brandy. Bottle and keep in the refrigerator.

Rose Toilet Water

2 large cups of fresh red rose petals
boiling water to cover
2 tablespoons gin or brandy

Pour the boiling water over the rose petals. Cover and leave to infuse at room temperature for twenty-four hours, then in the refrigerator for a further two days. Strain and add gin or brandy. Bottle and keep in the refrigerator.

Violet Water

Make according to the directions above for rose toilet water.
Similar toilet waters may be made from the leaves of lemon verbena or scented geranium, using the same recipe.

Lavender Toilet Water

Make according to the directions above for orange flower toilet water, substituting lavender flowers for the orange blossom.

Medika. Citrus

Those which are
called Median, or Persian,
or Cedromela, but in ye Latin
Citria, are knowne unto all,
for it is a tree that beares fruit
throughout ye whole yeare, one under
another. But the Apple it self, is
sommewhat long, wrinckled, resembling
gold in colour, smelling sweet with
heauinesse, hauing a seed like a peare.
It hath a facultie, being dranck in
wine, to resist poysons and subducere
alvum, & the decoction or iuce of it is a
collution for to make a sweet breath.
It is eaten especially by women [as a
remedy] against their lusting.

Dioscorides A.D. 60

DEODORANTS

Eating certain foods is reputed to influence our natural body odour. Meat eaters have a stronger body odour than those who live on vegetables. This does not necessarily mean that we should all become vegetarians, but that we should be moderate in our consumption of meat.

Natural deodorants do not prevent perspiration, but control perspiration odours by inhibiting the growth of micro-organisms which act on perspiration.

Herbal vinegars used as deodorants add a subdued perfume and possibly some antiseptic, according to the herbs used. Herbs suitable for making deodorant vinegars are rosemary, sage, lavender, spearmint, eau-de-cologne mint, thyme, yarrow, or any pungent herb which appeals.

To make herbal vinegar, take a quantity of herb, add a little apple cider vinegar and thoroughly bruise herb with a spoon or pestle. Place in a jar and pour over sufficient apple cider vinegar to just cover the bulk of the herb. Screw on the lid and leave to macerate a week to ten days on a sunny windowsill or in a warm place. When ready, strain off the vinegar. Bottle. Dilute before using as a deodorant — two tablespoons of water to one teaspoon of herbal vinegar.

After washing and drying under the arms, dab on the vinegar and allow to dry.

Diluted apple cider vinegar may be used on its own as a deodorant, if desired.

I find the following also very effective as a deodorant — one teaspoon of apple cider vinegar combined in a small bottle with two tablespoons of distilled wych hazel from the chemist.

To make a sage leaf infusion for a deodorant, take a handful of fresh sage leaves, pour over one cup of boiling water and leave to steep for twenty-four hours.

To use rosemary as a deodorant, make a strong decoction by placing leaves and soft twigs in a non-metal container and adding sufficient water to equal the quantity of herb. Bring slowly to the boil, simmer half an hour, then leave to cool before straining. After washing and drying under the arms, dab on some of the rosemary decoction and leave to dry on the skin.

Fresh lemon juice diluted in the ratio of one teaspoon of juice to two teaspoons of water may be dabbed under the arms and allowed to dry on the skin.

Take a handful of fresh parsley and put it through the juice extractor. After washing and drying under the arms dab on the green parsley juice liberally and allow to dry on.

Make an infusion of cleavers by taking six sprigs of the fresh herb and pouring over half a cup of boiling water. Allow to infuse twenty-four hours. After washing and drying under the arms, dab on the cleavers infusion and allow to dry on the skin.

Put a fresh lettuce leaf through the juice extractor and apply the juice liberally under the arms, leaving to dry on the skin.

Herbal Deodorant Stick

1½ tablespoons beeswax
½ tablespoon cocoa butter
1 tablespoon coconut oil
1 teaspoon oil of thyme
½ teaspoon rosemary oil
½ teaspoon lavender oil
3 drops castor oil

Melt the beeswax in a glass jar standing in hot water. Add the cocoa butter, and when it also has melted, put in the oils. Stir to mix thoroughly, then pour into a discarded deodorant-stick plastic case and leave to cool and set.

THE HANDS

The modern hazard for the hands, which replaces the damage done by hours of washing and scrubbing, is using detergent. Always wear protective gloves if you have to use detergent.

If your hands have been made dry and chapped by the excessive alkalinity of detergent, then you need to restore the acid mantle to your skin. Dilute one teaspoon of apple cider vinegar with two tablespoons of distilled water, rub into the hands and leave to dry on the skin.

The following hand cream made with lemon juice is also beneficial.

Lemon Hand Cream

1 teaspoon anhydrous lanolin (wool fat)
½ teaspoon apricot oil
½ teaspoon castor oil
1 teaspoon fresh lemon juice
½ teaspoon standard lemongrass
infusion (p. 39)

Melt the lanolin in a jar standing in hot water, add the oils, then the lemon juice, and lastly the lemongrass infusion. Remove from hot water bath, screw on lid and shake until cold.

Hand Oil
Very soothing for dry hands.

2 tablespoons apricot oil
1 tablespoon pumpkin oil

Combine in a bottle and shake.

Orange Flower Gel for the Hands

30 ml (1 fl oz) orange flower water (from the chemist)
½ teaspoon arrowroot
1 teaspoon coconut oil

Place the orange flower water in a jar standing in hot water and stir in the arrowroot powder. Add the coconut oil and keep stirring until the mixture thickens and turns clear. Screw the lid on the jar and shake well. Leave to cool, shaking occasionally.

Egg Creme for the Hands
Softening for the hands, legs and feet.

1 egg yolk
2 teaspoons lemon juice
¼ cup olive oil
¼ cup sunflower oil
6 drops lavender oil

Put the egg yolk and the lemon juice in the blender and whisk. Slowly add the oils and finally the lavender oil to perfume slightly. This will turn thick and creamy and keeps for a long time when refrigerated.

Elderflower Lotion
A light, soothing lotion, for softening the hands.

1 teaspoon standard elderflower infusion
(p. 39)
1 teaspoon almond milk
1 teaspoon apricot oil
½ teaspoon almond oil
½ teaspoon olive oil

Combine the ingredients and shake well.

Rose Hand Cream
This cream is soothing for dry hands and
is very suitable for rubbing into any dry
areas on the body and for softening hard
lines on the neck.

1 teaspoon beeswax
4 tablespoons rose toilet water (p. 113)
¼ teaspoon honey
4 tablespoons almond oil

Place the beeswax, almond oil and honey
in a jar standing in hot water, and stir
until they are melted together. Continue
stirring vigorously while pouring in the
rose toilet water. Remove the jar from
the water and stir well until the cream is
cool.

Dry Skin Hand Wash

Rub coconut oil into the hands, then wash them in warm water,
without using soap. Towel dry, leaving the skin soft and supple.

Oatmeal Hand Wash

For washing dirty hands, keep a small sprinkler jar filled with
powdered oatmeal (oatmeal flour) near the handbasin. Sprinkle a little
on to wet hands, rub until clean, then rinse.

The Nails

Smooth, well-groomed, healthy fingernails are an asset to one's general
appearance. Regular care is essential as fingernails deteriorate very
quickly if neglected. Problems such as splitting and brittleness usually
indicate a dietary deficiency. It is commonly known that sufficient
calcium is necessary for strong nails, but the mineral silica is equally
important. Helpful foods include barley, kelp, garlic, onion, parsley,
rice, chives, celery, lettuce, sunflower seed.

Dill and horsetail are the two herbs traditionally used to improve the fingernails. Both may be taken internally as teas and used externally as a finger bath. Make a strong infusion of one of the herbs for a finger bath and soak the finger tips in it ten to fifteen minutes. Massage a little olive or almond oil into the nails at night to help keep them supple. The old-fashioned method of buffing the nails with a chamois leather enhances their natural pink colouring and gives them a soft lustre. Rub a little oil into the cuticles to soften them, or heal any splits.

The oyle of wheat pressed forth between two plates of hot iron, healeth the chaps and chinks of the hands, feet, and fundament, which come of cold, making smooth the hands, face or any other part of the body.

Gerard's Herball
1597

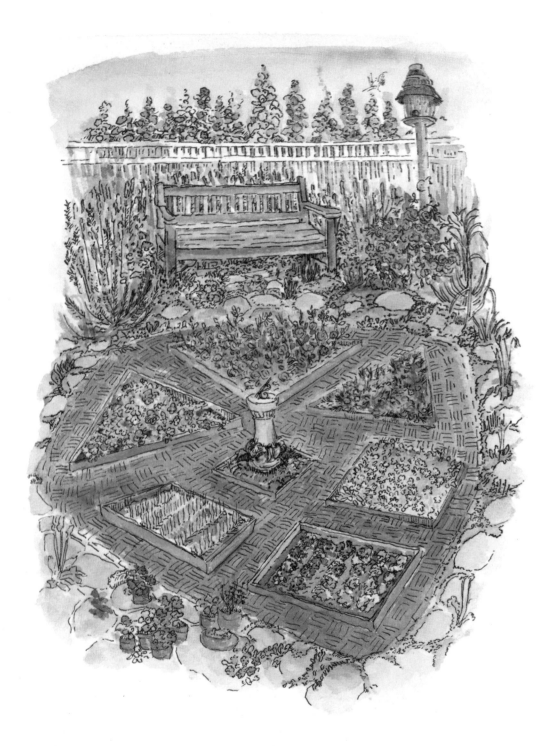

Remedy to Drive Away
Sweaty feet in a Person.

uadu - plant - of - the - fields
Eel - from - the - Canal

Warm in oil and smear both
feet therewith.

'The Papyrus Ebers'
1500 B.C.

THE FEET

Tired feet make a tired-looking face, so make some time to give them attention.

The old-fashioned foot bath, soaking the feet for ten to fifteen minutes, is a well-proven way of relaxing and reviving them. The herbs to use in a foot bath are any of the stimulant herbs such as rosemary, lavender, the mints, horsetail, yarrow or thyme. Make a double strength infusion of 60g herbs to 500 ml water (2 oz to 1 pint) and add this to a small bucket of warm water.

If you haven't time for a separate foot bath, rub rosemary oil or diluted apple cider vinegar into your feet, massaging for about five minutes, before you take a bath.

For dry skin on the feet, wash with a mixture of one tablespoon of bran and three tablespoons of strong chamomile infusion (about six level tablespoons chamomile flowers to one cup of water). Rinse, wipe dry, then use any of the hand creams or lotions to moisturise.

To soften extra hard skin around the soles of the feet or the backs of the heels, mix up equal quantities of castor oil and lemon juice and massage into the hard skin, or alternatively equal quantities of olive oil and apple cider vinegar. Keep rubbing until the excess oil is absorbed.

If you suffer from foot odour and excessive perspiration look to your diet and check that you are getting sufficient silica. Barley, kelp, horsetail tea, garlic, onion, parsley, lettuce, celery, are some of the silicon foods.

You should wear socks made from natural fibres because they breathe, whereas synthetics tend to encourage and emphasise perspiration. Change your socks and shoes daily, having several pairs of shoes so that you rotate them to give them a chance to air. If you must wear close-fitting shoes try sprinkling a little powdered dry chamomile flowers, peppermint leaves, pennyroyal or hyssop inside them. Wash your feet daily with an infusion of cleavers. Air your feet as frequently as possible by going barefoot.

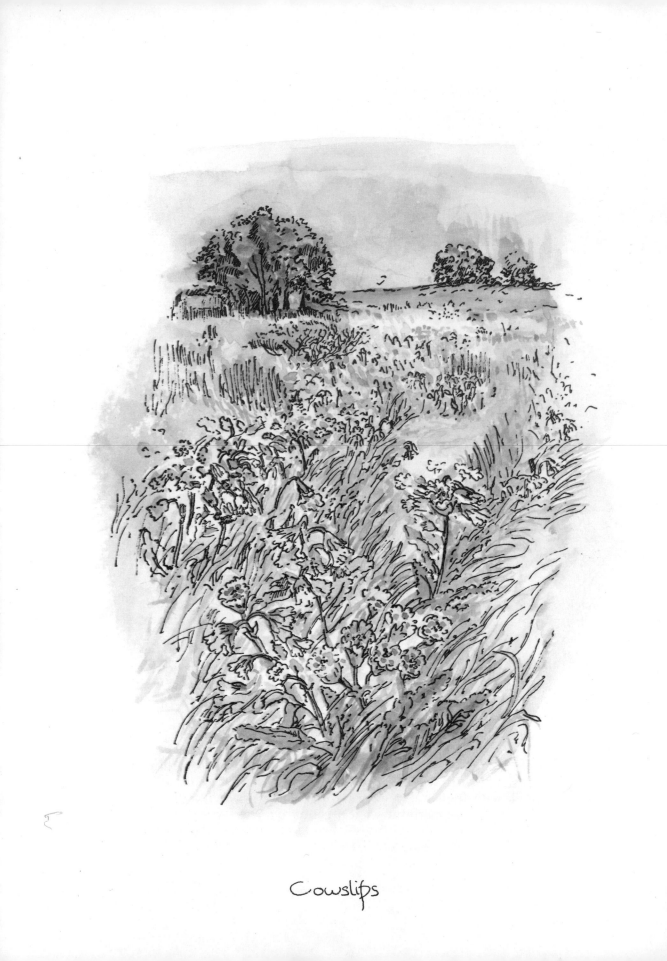

Cowslips

CARE OF THE BODY OUTDOORS

Out in the Sun

Over-exposure to the sun prematurely ages the skin and in hot climates can cause skin cancer. On the other hand, a moderate amount of sunshine increases the circulation and ensures sufficient manufacture of vitamin D. It helps to keep us healthy, so don't fear the sun, but treat it with respect. Sunbathe in moderation.

Oils to use to soften the skin after sunbathing are sesame, olive, coconut and apricot.

Remember, too, that swimming in chlorinated or salt water is drying to the skin, so be sure to rinse your body thoroughly in fresh water and rub on a little oil after a day at the beach or the pool.

Herbs for Sunburn

If you do get sunburned there are many simple lotions you can make to soothe and cool the skin.

Cucumber juice made in the juice extractor with an unpeeled cucumber, or a mild infusion (p. 39) of lettuce leaves, chamomile, elderflower or cowslip are all effective remedies. The juice of the houseleek pressed from the fresh leaf is very anti-inflammatory and soothing to the skin.

Herbs to Protect Skin from the Sun

There are many herbs, juices and natural products which keep the skin from darkening, burning and freckling. However, you will still need to be moderate in exposure to the sun. If you burn easily or have other detrimental reactions to too much sunshine, wear a hat. This will have the added benefit of shading your eyes from the glare and preventing squinting and crowsfeet. A long-sleeved cotton blouse is protective for arms and shoulders.

Almond Oil

A little rubbed into the skin helps prevent freckles and sunburn.

Cucumber Juice

Used as a skin freshener soothes and whitens the skin. You may prefer to use a moisturising lotion containing the juice as an ingredient (see Index).

Cowslip Infusion

May be made and used in the same manner as elderflower water (see below).

Buttermilk

Buttermilk keeps the skin white, used on its own if you have oily skin, or made into a lotion if you have dry skin.

Elderflower Water

Make a mild infusion (p. 39), steep, then strain and bottle. This herb has an age-old reputation for keeping the skin white and protecting it from the effects of the sun. Use elderflower water first thing in the morning, or at any time during the day prior to going out in the sun. Use a moisturising lotion containing elderflower infusion as an ingredient (see Index).

To Whiten a V-Neckline

Dresses with collars and revers, or a V-neckline, encourage concentration of the sunlight on a small area of skin and increase sunburn, reddening and veining of the neck and chest.

Apply a lotion of elderflower water (above) and almond oil to this vulnerable area, to reduce redness and veins, to whiten and soothe.

Dealing with Insects

Herbal Insect Repellents

One very happy effect of using herbal and natural lotions and oils is that the mosquitoes usually don't like the taste of you.

Oil of Lavender or Citronella

These are well-known insect repellents but don't use them outdoors without adequate protection from cotton clothing as they make some people's skin photosensitive (sensitive to sun and light).

Lemon Balm, Pennyroyal and Basil

Fresh leaves rubbed on the skin repel insects, and should you have been bitten before thinking of applying them, they will relieve itching when bruised and rubbed into a bite.

Elderflower

Disliked by mosquitoes and flies. Use elderflower water (p. 126) rubbed on the skin.

Insect Bite Soothers

Hyssop, Plantain, Rosemary and Yarrow

Leaves applied to bites and stings are soothing.

Cornflower

An infusion (p. 39) takes the itch out of insect bites.

EXERCISE

To keep the body fit and beautiful, with the movable joints flexible and all the muscles toned and resilient so that normal physical exertion does not produce fatigue or pain, requires regular exercise in some form or another. This may be done incidentally through everyday activities, or by playing sport, or by following a set pattern of exercises.

The human being was created as a functional entity. Every part is meant to be used. Neglect any part, discontinue using it, and degeneration will set in. This is true not only of the body, but of the mind. Hence, to remain fit and alert, regular exercise and activity are necessary. However, remembering the balance that is inherent in nature, to over-exercise and overwork to the point of exhaustion will equally promote degeneration. Moderation is the key.

There are many kinds of exercise programmes currently in use throughout the world. Some are traditional movements which originated centuries ago and have been passed down through successive generations. Two examples are Indian yoga and Chinese "shadow-boxing".

Other programmes are modern and up-to-the-minute routines based on scientific data and technological checking instruments for pulse, blood pressure and so on. There are exercises which were formulated to ensure the physical fitness of the armed forces, others to bring to perfection the performance of athletes, while there are less arduous systems for the layman.

For those of you who wish to follow a formal exercise programme, I have included the following "Family Exercise Programme" with the kind permission of the Division of Recreation and Sport in conjunction with the Institute for Fitness, Research and Training, and the South Australian Women's Keep Fit Association Inc.

Family Exercise Programme

Do the following exercises at least three times a week but preferably daily — each daily session taking between ten and fifteen minutes.

Whenever you exercise it is important to warm-up, to ease into the exercise routine gradually. Stretching (mobilising) exercises are among the easiest and most pleasant. The first three are examples of the many mobilising exercises.

This programme attempts to provide a guide to exercises that are necessary to maintain adequate joint mobility, muscle function and posture. It is important to realise that a programme such as this cannot fulfil everybody's specific needs. The exercises are presented as a guide only, for many variations and progressions can be used to suit individual needs. (Note that all the exercises are suitable for both men and women.)

Precautions:

1. If you are in any doubt about your health; have a chronic joint-muscle problem; any cardiovascular problem; or are over 35 years of age, it is prudent to consult a doctor (or in some cases, a physiotherapist) before starting to exercise.

2. When embarking on a physical activity that you have not done before or have not done for some time, you must start very gently and progress very gradually to allow your body time to adapt to the unaccustomed demands (i.e. to avoid undue stiffness and soreness).

3. If any particular exercise troubles you (e.g. aggravates your "bad back") do not do that exercise and seek further advice. (Problems should not be expected as these exercises have been selected because they are "safe" if performed correctly.)

4. DO NOT DO ANY OF THE EXERCISES WITH BOUNCING, JERKING, FLINGING OR UNCONTROLLED MOVEMENTS. All your movements should be controlled, smooth and rhythmical.

5. Breathe naturally and avoid holding your breath.

6. Relax the muscles being used after each repetition of an exercise.

The Exercises

S.P. = Starting Position

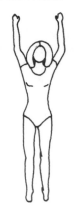

1. *Stretch*
S.P.: Standing. Extend your arms above your head, breathing in. Stretch up, reaching as high as you can. Relax, lower arms and repeat.

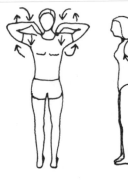

2. *Shoulder Rotation*
S.P.: Standing, back straight. To rotate lift the shoulders, press them back, down and around. Relax. Repeat 6 forward rotations then 6 backward rotations.

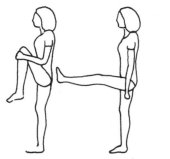
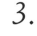

3. *Knee Lift*
S.P.: Standing. Keeping your back straight, draw the knee to the chest. Return to the standing position. Repeat 5-6 times using alternate legs. As a progression start the exercise as before, then stretch the leg forwards before returning it to the floor.

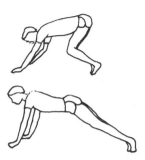

4. *Caterpillar (General Exercise)*
S.P.: Standing. Bend your knees, drop your hands to the floor, and walk forward on your hands until your body is straight.
Do not let the back sag. Walk your hands back, then stand. Relax. Repeat 5-6 times.

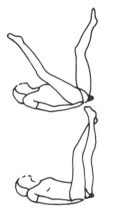

5. *Scissors (Inner/outer Thigh)*
S.P.: Lying on the back, hands beneath the buttocks. Raise legs together above the hips. Part the legs sideways. Bring them back together in a scissor motion, crossing the legs alternatively. Repeat 10 times, breathing regularly.

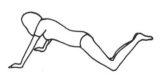

6. *Arm Strengthening Exercise*
A. Basic Exercise — Knee push up.
S.P.: Lying on your stomach, knees bent. Place your hands at shoulder level. Keeping the head and shoulders down, with the arms lift the whole body to the knees in one movement. Lower the body to the floor in the same way. Relax. Repeat 5-10 times.
B. For those who are unable to keep the body straight do the following variation.

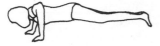

S.P.: On all fours. Move weight forward on to your hands. Lower chest to the floor and press up.

C. For those who can do the basic exercise correctly and find it easy, progress to a full push up.

7. *Upper Back Exercise*

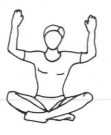

S.P.: Sitting, preferably cross-legged. Breathe in, straighten the spine, stretch up, lift the arms at the sides to shoulder height and press them backwards keeping the head in line with the back. Lower arms, relax forward, breathe out. Repeat 5-10 times.

8. *Abdominal Exercise*

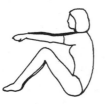

A. Basic Exercise: S.P.: Sitting, knees bent with the feet flat on the floor, arms stretched forward. With rounded shoulders and the chin tucked down, lean back to the floor. Curl the chin onto the chest and sit up.
Repeat as many times as possible up to 20. Breathe naturally and avoid holding your breath.

B. If you are unable to return to the sitting position: Start the exercise as above but only lean back sufficiently far to allow yourself to return to the sitting position.

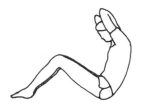

C. Progression: If you find the basic exercise easy try these arm position variations:
  (i) fold your arms across your midriff or
  (ii) clasp your hands behind your head.

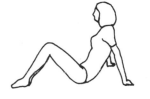

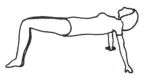

9. *Body Lift (General Exercise)*
S.P.: Sitting, knees bent. With the weight resting on the hands lift the hips off the floor until the body is straight. Lower body to the floor. Repeat 5-10 times.

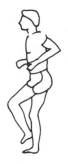

10. *Jogging/Skipping*
Starting with 30 seconds to 1 minute gradually build up to 3-5 minutes of the following suggestions:
  (i) Skipping; with or without a rope.
  (ii) Jogging on the spot; combinations of swinging legs to the side, kicking forward, heels up, knees up.
  (iii) Jumping; little jumps, feet apart to the side and together, both feet from side to side, forward jumps etc.
CAUTION: Make sure you ease your heel to the ground after each step, when jogging or skipping on the spot.

Points to Note

1. If an exercise programme is to have any beneficial effect the programme must be performed regularly. The effects of exercise fade rapidly when the necessary stimulus is removed. Remember that habits are acquired over a period of time.

2. Try to take as much incidental exercise as possible e.g. Walk or cycle instead of using the car. Use stairs instead of the lift etc. Simply BE MORE ACTIVE.

3. Most people find it easier to maintain the commitment to increasing their physical activity by exercising with a group. Round up some friends to join you.

4. Individuals who are sedentary need to do more aerobic exercises (rhythmic endurance exercises to condition the cardio-vascular system) such as jogging, brisk walking, cycling, swimming and skipping, in addition to the calisthenic exercises described in this programme.

To have a "training effect", that is, to bring about improvements in cardio-vascular function, aerobic exercises require the heart to beat fairly fast, roughly between 65 per cent and 80 per cent of the maximum rate of which the heart is capable.

A handy formula for this is: $(220 - \text{your age}) \times \dfrac{75}{100}$ e.g. $220 - 35 \text{ years} \times 75\% = 139$ bpm.

Learn to take your pulse so that you know how hard you (via your heart) are working. Aerobic exercise needs to be moderately strenuous, "somewhat hard" is an apt subjective description, but it does not need to be exhausting. A recommended amount of aerobic exercise is three fifteen to twenty-five-minute bouts a week (less than 1 per cent of the total time in the week, less than 2 per cent of one's time awake!)

5. The calisthenic programme is a useful warm-up to any aerobic work, or sports training.

A HEALTHY DIET

Emotions Surrounding Food

The whole subject of food is interwoven with a variety of emotions. Take, for example, its use for both reward and punishment in private life by the parent who says to the child, "Do as I say and I'll give you a nice sweetie", or "You'll go to bed without your dinner", or in public life by the State Banquet for the privileged as opposed to the one-time prisoner on bread and water.

Food has long been a symbol of social status — as witnessed in the caviar and champagne syndrome, or in the trendy following of every new fad. For centuries eating has been used as a means of celebration, from the upper-class orgy of the past to the present day middle-class: "Let's go out to dinner and celebrate".

It has long been regarded as a token of friendship and goodwill to share your food with another human being.

Food selection and habits identify "nations". They may be seen as a symbol of security and order in society, for example, the regular Sunday roast dinner. On the other hand they may be a sign of personal disorder when food is used as a retreat and comfort in stress by the worrier who feels the need constantly to eat and drink.

It is necessary to cut through all these emotions to see that food is our vital link with the natural order of the world and our sure way to good health.

Thoughtful Selection of Foods

Nature has been bountiful, so there is an infinite variety of foods from which to choose, and we should all make as wide and varied a selection as possible to ensure a steady supply of every type of necessary nutriment.

It would not only be boring mentally, but restrictive and unbalanced for the body, to choose one rigid set pattern of food as "ideal" to eat year in and year out. It should be borne in mind, too, that any one food or drink taken to excess may be harmful, no matter how health-giving it is in moderation. Vary your choice of food to delight the palate and nourish the body. Select from natural, basic foods like vegetables, fruit, grains, nuts, meats, eggs, cheeses, as far as possible from foods grown in your own region to ensure freshness — but there is no need to be a faddist about it. If you wish to add piquancy or sweetness to your foods, do so by the addition of herbs rather than with quantities of salt, sugar or synthetic flavourings. It seems only commonsense to be moderate in the use of sugar and salt. The palate adapts itself very quickly to sweetness and bitterness, and it is interesting how nasty both these products taste in large amounts when you are not used to them.

Follow the natural changing seasons in your eating pattern. In the hot weather tend more toward the cooling foods and drinks. Salads can be made from an extensive range of raw young vegetables. The old standby of lettuce, tomato and cucumber is only one of many possibilities. Beans, peas, zucchini, capsicum, endive, mustard and cress, onions, cauliflower, cabbage, beetroot, as well as mushrooms, carrot tops, dandelion, chicory, alfalfa, mint and watercress may all be eaten raw. You can probably think of many other examples, as this is not an exhaustive list.

It should not be necessary to be constantly stimulating yourself with drinks of tea, coffee or cocoa. I think we have forgotten that the purpose of drinking is to quench the thirst. Drink water, vegetable and fruit juices, remembering that the extremes of ice-cold, or conversely red-hot, drinks are not kind to the stomach or the digestion. Leave out the fizzy drinks and the cordials which are virtually liquid sugar. Besides, they tend to increase the thirst.

Eat your daily bread and unprocessed cereal, and some fish or the lighter cuts of meat. In the winter tend more toward the warming foods like grains and pulses, dried fruits and nuts, as well as plenty of vegetables. Keep your meat consumption proportionate to that of vegetables in the ratio of one part meat to at least three parts vegetables.

Shortcook your vegetables, that is, cook them gently in a heavy saucepan with a lid, the base having been lightly greased or oiled to prevent sticking, thus eliminating the need for water. The vegetables are done when crisp but chewable, not soggy, and there is no vegetable water to strain off, pouring the vitamins down the kitchen sink.

Make side salads from raw, fresh, winter vegetables, including celery, broccoli, leeks, parsnips, turnips, turnip tops and so on. Make bean casseroles. Don't forget there is a wide choice of grains like oats, buckwheat, millet, rye and barley, as well as wheat flour to make into cereals, pies, bread or scones.

A healthy diet should include sufficient fibre from vegetables and grains to keep the digestive tract working to digest your food properly, allow absorption of its nutriments and finally to eliminate the waste through regular bowel movements several times a day.

Junk Foods

Junk foods consist primarily of sugar, artificial colouring and flavouring, preservatives, fats, bleached flour and over-processed grains or cereals. They are unbalanced and non-nutritious. Yet this kind of food is very often seen as a reward, particularly by children and misguided relatives and friends, and is promoted by television advertising. It amounts to a confidence trick on the taste buds.

How boring to have everything approximately the same sweetness and flavour, when nature has provided us with an amazing variety of tastes and tangs to enjoy. If we deaden our responses by constant artificial sweetness, then we become stultified and negative about our choice of food. It follows that the metabolism becomes upset and we live deprived lives nutritionally, no matter how affluent we may be in other ways.

Junk food is a twentieth century innovation, resulting from the rapid increase in technology and a desire to provide cheap food on a massive scale for large populations; an ambition which has gone too far in one rigid direction. It is necessary now to swing the pendulum back, to get away from the artificial or synthetic, and return to fresh, natural foods, to the benefit of our present and future health.

Prior to the twentieth century, the normal diet consisted of a variety of the basic foods. Dietary fibre, now hailed as a radical new discovery, was an ordinary part of daily eating. People naturally ate high-fibre diets, obtaining vegetable fibre from the garden and grain fibre in unprocessed cereals and flours.

If we generally avoid eating chocolates, lollies, commercially produced biscuits, cake and ice-cream, fizzy drinks, cordials, white bread, potato chips, quick snack products and instant breakfast foods, then at those times when it is socially prudent to eat them, we can do so with impunity, knowing our well-cared-for body can handle anything in small amounts.

However, one should not have to be self-righteous about food; just use commonsense.

Instant Meals

If food is our best preventive medicine, as I believe it is, then how foolish we are if we don't put some thought and time into its selection and presentation. Nevertheless there are occasions when we are busy or need a break from routine and a meal has to be put quickly on the table. So many people take the line of least resistance these days and head for the commercially produced instant meal, which consists so often of dead food, stale and over-cooked, and tending to the cheaper, non-nutritious ingredients like sugar, salt and white flour, and all those cooked and re-cooked fats for frying up rissoles, chips and chickens. Eat too much of this type of food and you will soon lack the energy to get on to preparing your own.

When in a hurry or a lazy mood, it is surely not difficult to open a loaf of grain bread, a packet of camembert cheese, or some dried fruit. It takes only a few minutes to boil an egg, collate an original salad from whatever fresh vegetables are immediately available, or pick up a piece of raw fruit. Fresh fish rolled in wheat germ is cooked in no time in a lightly oiled frypan.

Use a little imagination and a meal can be served quickly and without fuss, and it will be a positively contributing meal which will carry you on in health and energy.

A Varied and Sustaining Diet

Eat foods that are compatible with your metabolism; in other words, those that agree with you. Avoid foods that disagree, for example those that cause flatulence, nausea, or just a general feeling of "I wish I hadn't eaten that". Your own body will tell you what is good for you. Everyone is different, so it would be a mistake to say there is one ideal diet suitable for every person.

Every day you should make a choice from each of the following categories:
1. Vegetables.
2. Grains.
3. Pulses (dried peas, beans and lentils); meats and fish; eggs; cheese.
4. Fruit, nuts; seeds.

As far as it is practical, make a varied selection according to what is in season, the climate, and the location in which you live. There are a dozen different vegetables, as many fruits, and several choices of grains to keep your diet interesting and to ensure a cross-section of all the different nutriments necessary to health.

The three basic meals per day should be sufficiently nourishing to carry you through from one to the next, without becoming excessively hungry or fatigued. I am not advocating that you over-eat. If your food is fresh and nutritious, you won't need to eat vast quantities in order to satisfy your appetite. It is important to remember, too, that if you don't feel like eating at a particular time, you shouldn't eat.

Obviously, to be sustaining, breakfast must consist of something other than a quick coffee and toast, or a processed cereal. Many people feel they can't face breakfast, probably because they ate too much or too late the night before. Nervous tension and the inability to relax play a role here, too, so there could be several factors to look into.

Millet, oat or bran porridge will all help to set you up for the day ahead, as will muesli, preferably made by you. To make your own muesli use any combination of ingredients like bran, soaked oats, barley kernels or unroasted buckwheat, plus crushed nuts or sunflower or sesame seeds, a little dried fruit, and raw fresh fruit such as grated apple, any of the berry fruits, or orange, lemon or apricot juice. Some people may prefer cooked pulses or a boiled egg. It is a matter of personal preference.

A substantial lunch, including plenty of vegetables, either cooked or raw, eliminates the four o'clock fatigue as the working day nears completion, and prevents the desperate hunger in the evening that makes people gorge themselves.

It is a pity that our meal times are so often rigidly set by commercial considerations, and people are obliged to eat when they are not ready to do so or when they are over-hungry. Dinner at night ideally should be a moderate meal, but this is not always possible, and if it has to be the main meal of the day, relax and enjoy it — but not too late at night, so that your body has time to get on to the work of digestion several hours before you retire to bed. Remember:

- Freshness
- Variety
- Moderation
- Enjoyment

These should be the criteria by which you select your daily food, rather than fretting over how many vitamins and minerals are being consumed with every mouthful.

Vitamins and Minerals

Vitamins and vitamin pills have been so over-emphasised during the last few years that people have been led to believe they are "magic bullets" for health. Unfortunately, this is a modern fallacy. There is no one isolated factor which will promote or maintain health. Everything in nature interacts, relates and balances in an intricate and delicate equipoise. An over-enthusiastic intake of vitamins and minerals may lead to an over-emphasis of one element which may in turn cause a deficiency in another. Most people do not realise that most vitamins and minerals need a catalyst or a complement to make them freely available to the human body, that they do not work on their own. Consequently, to depend on vitamin and other tablets in an endeavour to make up a dietary deficiency is a hit and miss approach. In natural foods, nature has provided the necessary balance of complementary vitamins, minerals and other elements to make them available to the body and beneficial to health, therefore it seems more sensible to assure your daily intake by a thoughtful selection of foods.

Weight Problems

It is unwise to embark on crash diets or grossly unbalanced diets which stipulate over-eating one nutriment like protein, while depriving the body of a normal range of food. It is far better to lose weight slowly, to allow the body to make a gradual adjustment, particularly the skin, which can become flabby because it has not had time to shrink after a rapid weight loss. Eat a balanced diet, but eat less overall. Concentrate on raw foods whenever possible. Cut out all unnecessary eating. When you feel like heading for the kitchen to

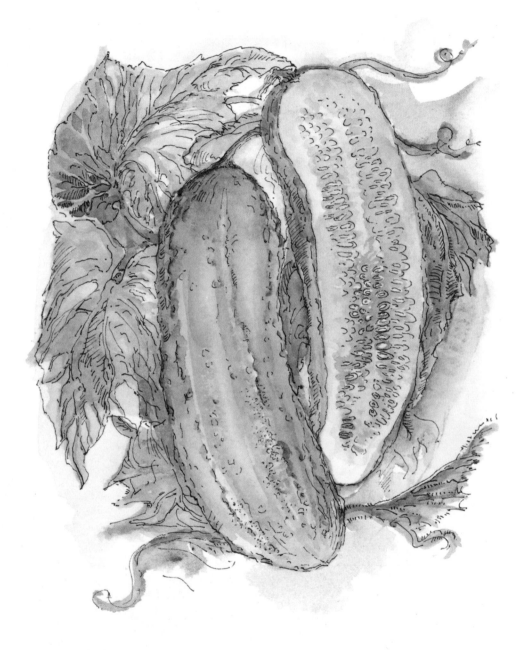

comfort yourself, get busy on some absorbing work or hobby and you'll forget the desire for extra food.

Omit all junk food. Don't overwork and make sure you are getting adequate rest at night. Don't overdrink. Drink when thirsty. Take sensible exercise. For the average person without any serious medical problem, this should be all that is necessary to ensure a steady, healthy weight loss.

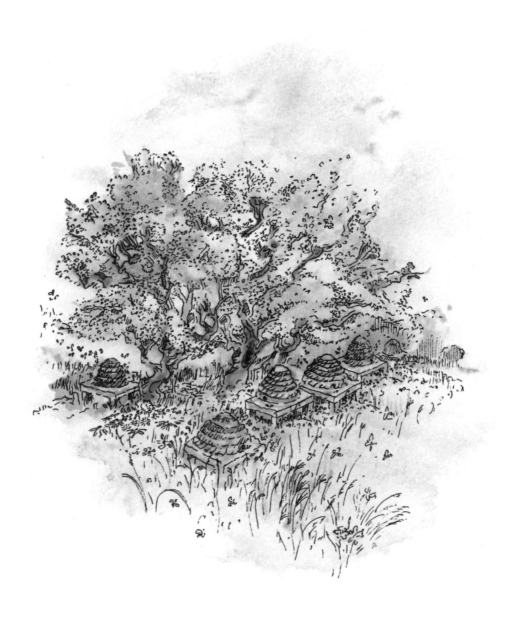

PART V

THE HAIR:
Care of the Hair
Conditioning the Hair
Herbal Shampoos
Herbal Rinses
Setting Lotions
Hair Problems

CARE OF THE HAIR

The condition of the hair is usually a good indication of the state of your general health. Feel just a bit off-colour and it is surprising how quickly the hair loses its sheen and body. You must ensure that you are eating a healthy, balanced diet to have healthy, beautiful hair. Many dietary factors are involved in good hair health, some of which are vitamin B complex, vitamin A, calcium, silica, iron, zinc, protein and unsaturated oils or fatty acids.

Although diet is the foundation of beautiful hair, the way you care for your hair is important too. You should brush your hair regularly with a pure bristle brush to shake out dust and to condition it naturally. Wash your hair only when necessary, probably once a week, as too-frequent shampooing can over-stimulate the scalp and induce oiliness, so that you have oily hair near the scalp and dry, brittle ends. Conditioning the hair before washing it will take care of dry ends, but a shampoo which cleans without stripping the hair will eliminate the need for pre-conditioning.

Choice of shampoo is important because so many commercial shampoos are largely detergent (similar to dishwashing liquid, which is very alkaline and drying). Shampoos can strip the oil from the hair and the scalp, causing the hair to be unmanageable and out of condition. Incidentally, this drying-out of the scalp carries over to the face and may cause or increase facial dryness.

Hair is so very individual that it is not always easy to find a shampoo that perfectly suits it, and after a while the satisfactory shampoo may seem to have lost its suitability. This is because the hair and scalp respond to changes in diet, health and the environment. Using herbs it is possible to create an individual shampoo which can be varied as often as necessary.

Always wet hair thoroughly with warm water before applying shampoo, as it is a concentrated liquid. You must be careful to rinse out the shampoo thoroughly before drying your hair.

Diluted lemon juice or cider vinegar, using about one tablespoon to five cups of water, makes an acid rinse which restores the natural pH balance to the hair.

To avoid putting strain on the hair when wet, comb it layer by layer, starting with the underneath hair and working up to the top layer. Any tangles are easily eliminated by this method of combing. Don't brush wet hair or you'll split the ends and pull it out by the roots at an unnatural rate.

You should always keep your brushes and combs scrupulously clean as a regular part of hair care. Wash them in a diluted rosemary decoction to eliminate any build-up of grease and to give them a delightfully fresh smell.

To make rosemary decoction, place equal quantities of fresh rosemary and water in a non-metal container, and simmer gently for about half an hour. Strain.

Marshmallow
[Althea Officinalis]

The juice of Mallows boiled in old oil, takes away roughness of the skin, scurf, or dry scabs in the head, or other parts, if they be anointed with the decoction, and preserves the hair from falling off.

Culpeper 1653

CONDITIONING THE HAIR

Pre-Conditioning

If the hair is brittle or has split ends it is wise to pre-condition it before shampooing. Coconut oil, olive oil or castor oil are all suitable. Rub a small quantity into the scalp and hair and wrap your head in a warm wet towel for thirty minutes, putting a shower cap over the towel to keep the warmth in.

Shampoo and give a final rinse with vinegar or lemon in the water.

For dry hair that is tangly when wet, pre-condition with a few drops of rosemary oil or half and half rosemary and lavender. Rub well in about half an hour before shampooing.

Conditioning the Hair After Shampooing

If you feel it is necessary to condition the hair after shampooing, take one to two drops of oil, rub between the palms of the hands and lightly apply over your wet hair. Rosemary oil, lavender oil, or a combination of both, are very suitable.

For brittle hair, mix two-thirds rosemary oil with one-third olive oil, and apply in the same manner.

Henna Shampoo

1½ tablespoons Henna

½ teaspoon powdered Borax

1 cake finely shredded Soap

½ pint boiling water

Simmer slowly, strain and set in pots.

To use : After washing the hair, put on henna shampoo. Leave on five minutes. Do this three times, then rinse.

My Great-Grandmother's recipe
circa 1910

HERBAL SHAMPOOS

Basic Herbal Shampoo Recipe

1 cup herbal infusion
(see basic recipe p. 39 and take
your choice of herb from the lists below)
2 caps or small teaspoons saponified
coconut oil (see p. 176)
1 teaspoon glycerin

Combine in a plastic bottle and shake. An alternative method of making the herbal shampoo is to omit the glycerin and simply add the 2 small teaspoons of saponified coconut oil to the cup of water used to brew the herb of your choice.

The hair herbs may be used individually or in any combination you prefer.

Herbs for Shampoos for All Hair Types

Nettle

One of the best known of the hair herbs which is stimulating to the circulation of the scalp and gently cleansing to the hair. Make a weak infusion of the dried herb and steep thirty minutes. Strain and use.

Rosemary

Another popular hair herb particularly for use on dark hair as it emphasises the deeper shades of hair colour. Boil three tablespoons of fresh herb in one cup of water ten minutes. Steep fifteen minutes. Strain and use. It leaves the hair delightfully fragrant.

Southernwood

A cleansing, antiseptic herb with a fresh, pungent scent. It keeps the scalp healthy and stimulates the hair follicles. Make a decoction by chopping up four tablespoons of fresh herb and simmering it gently in one cup of water for five to ten minutes. Strain and cool sufficiently before using.

Burdock

A herb which is soothing and healing to any scalp irritation while being cleansing to the hair. Soak one teaspoon of chopped, dried root in one cup of cold water for several hours. Bring gently to the boil, then strain. Cool sufficiently before using.

Parsley

A herb that is healing to scalp conditions while stimulating the hair. It balances the sebaceous glands. Take two tablespoons of freshly chopped parsley leaves and boil them five minutes in one cup of water. Strain and cool before using.

Elderflower

A gentle stimulant to the hair as well as being anti-inflammatory and healing to the scalp. Make a weak infusion, steeping for half an hour. Strain and use.

Lemon Verbena

A cleansing, fragrant herb which is a pore stimulant. Make a mild infusion of the fresh or dried herb, steeping half an hour. Strain and use.

Catmint

A herb which promotes growth and adds a delightful shine to the hair. Make a mild infusion, steeping for half an hour. Strain and use.

Emollient Herbs for Shampoos for Dry Hair

Marshmallow

A well known hair herb which is mucilaginous so is softening and conditioning in its effect. Simmer half a tablespoon of chopped dried root in one cup of water for half an hour. Strain and cool before using.

Comfrey

Use either the leaf or the root of this herb. If your hair is particularly dry, the mucilaginous root will be more conditioning. A healing and cooling herb for irritated scalp conditions. Make a weak infusion of the leaves, or a mild decoction of the rootstock. Strain and cool before use.

Chamomile

A herb that is anti-inflammatory and healing to scalp irritations. A tonic for fair hair as it has a lightening effect with yellow highlights. Make a weak infusion, steeping for half an hour. Strain and use.

Quince

A very old hair tonic is made from the peel of ripe quinces. Boil the peel of half a quince in one cup of water for ten to fifteen minutes. Strain and cool before use.

Red Clover

A gently cleansing herb. Boil one teaspoon of the dried flowers in one cup of water for five minutes. Strain and cool before using.

Astringent Herbs for Shampoos for Oily Hair

Horsetail

A cleansing herb which stimulates the growth of the hair. Soak half a tablespoon in a cup of water for two hours, then simmer it for ten minutes. Leave to steep off the heat for fifteen minutes. Strain and cool before use.

Sage

A herb for dark hair as it enhances the deeper colour tones. Make a mild infusion of freshly chopped sage leaves and steep two hours. Strain and use.

Thyme

A cleansing and tonic herb which imparts a lovely fresh fragrance to the hair. Infuse three tablespoons of fresh herb in a cup of boiling water. Steep for twenty-four hours. Strain and use.

Yarrow

A refreshing, cleansing herb which is a tonic for the hair. Make a mild infusion of the fresh leaves, steeping for an hour. Strain and use.

Lemon Balm

A gently cleansing herb which imparts a spicy lemon scent to the hair. Add some lemon peel if you have fair hair and wish to enhance the fragrance. Make a mild infusion of the fresh leaves, steeping for half an hour. Strain and use.

Lemongrass

Another cleansing, lemon-scented herb. Make an infusion of half a tablespoon of dried chopped leaves to one cup of boiling water. Steep half an hour. Strain and use.

Maidenhair
(Asplenium Ruta Muraria)

The lye made thereof is singularly
good to cleanse the head from
scurf, and from dry and running sores;
stays the shedding or falling of the hair,
and causes it to grow thick, fair, and
well-coloured; for which purpose boil it
in wine, putting some smallage seed
thereto, and afterwards some oil.

Culpeper 1653

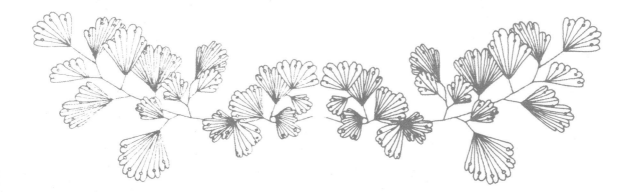

Fagus & Ilex, being both a kinde
of Oake, worke the like effects,
but ye barck of the roote of the Ilex
being sod in water till it becomnes
tender and rotten, & being layd on
for a whole night, doth dye the
haire black, being first made cleane
with Cimolian earth ....

Oak Galls. They doe also make the
haire black, being macerated in vinegar,
                              or water.
    Dioscorides
            A.D. 60

HERBAL RINSES

Make a herbal infusion (p. 39) and, using a catch-bowl, pour the liquid several times over the wet hair after shampooing.

To make dark hair shiny

Parsley, sage or rosemary in a weak infusion (p. 39).

To make fair hair shiny

Chamomile, yarrow or marigold in a weak infusion (p. 39).

For white hair

Make a strong infusion (p. 39) of blue cornflowers.

To highlight dark hair

Diluted lemon juice.

To lighten fair hair

Make a strong infusion (p. 39) of chamomile, steeping two hours at least.

To darken dark hair

Make a strong infusion (p. 39) of sage, steeping overnight. If you wish, add some black tea.

   If your hair is in good condition you could apply the above herbs as a gel by thickening a strong infusion with arrowroot powder, or quince or flaxseed gel (pp. 41, 180) and leaving on the hair for half an hour. Then rinse thoroughly. It would be wise to do a patch first to estimate the effect on your hair.

Generally speaking, herbal rinses or gels must be used regularly to show any marked effect, as herbs work slowly, not drastically.

WAVING LOTION

One teaspoon of glycerine mixed gradually with six tablespoons of elderflower water or rosewater, one teaspoon of rectified spirit, and half a teaspoon of ammonia.

My Great-Grandmother's recipe
circa 1910

SETTING LOTIONS

Quince Setting Lotion

A well known old recipe for setting lotion is made from quince seeds taken from the ripened fruit. Soak one teaspoon of seeds in a cup of cold water overnight to make a gel.

Flaxseed Setting Lotion

Flaxseed may also be used, but you will need to soak two tablespoons of seed in one cup of water until a gel forms.

Rosemary Setting Lotion

Make a decoction of rosemary by simmering two tablespoons of herb in two and a half cups of water for five minutes. Allow to steep until cool. Strain and add a few drops of rosemary oil if desired. Suitable for dark hair.

Sage Setting Lotion

Make an infusion of one teaspoon of leaves to one and a quarter cups of boiling water. Steep until cold. A variation for dark hair.

Chamomile Setting Lotion

Make as for rosemary with the addition of a little chopped lemon peel. For fair hair.

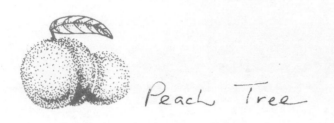

Peach Tree

If the kernels be bruised
and boiled in vinegar, until
they become thick, and
applied to the head, it marvell-
ously makes the hair to grow
again upon bald places, or
where it is too thin.

Culpeper 1653

HAIR PROBLEMS

Slow-growing Hair

Herbs to Promote Growth of the Hair

If the hair is cared for regularly and correctly it should grow at a normal, healthy rate. If it needs a boost, it is a matter of stimulating the circulation and the nerve supply to the scalp. Brushing the hair with a natural bristle brush with your head bent down is a simple way to begin.

There are many herbs which help stimulate the scalp, particularly when applied as lotions to the hair roots. When applying herbal lotions, massage, knead or vibrate — don't rub the scalp or you'll lose hair.

Nettle Lotion

Make a tea or a weak infusion of dried nettle leaves, massaging a little into the scalp several times a week to stimulate circulation.

Southernwood Lotion

Make a mild infusion (p. 39). Massage into the hair several times a week, or use as a final rinse after washing the hair.

Parsley Lotion

Use the seeds or the leaves to make an infusion, or juice the leaves and apply the green lotion to the scalp, leaving for about an hour before a shampoo.

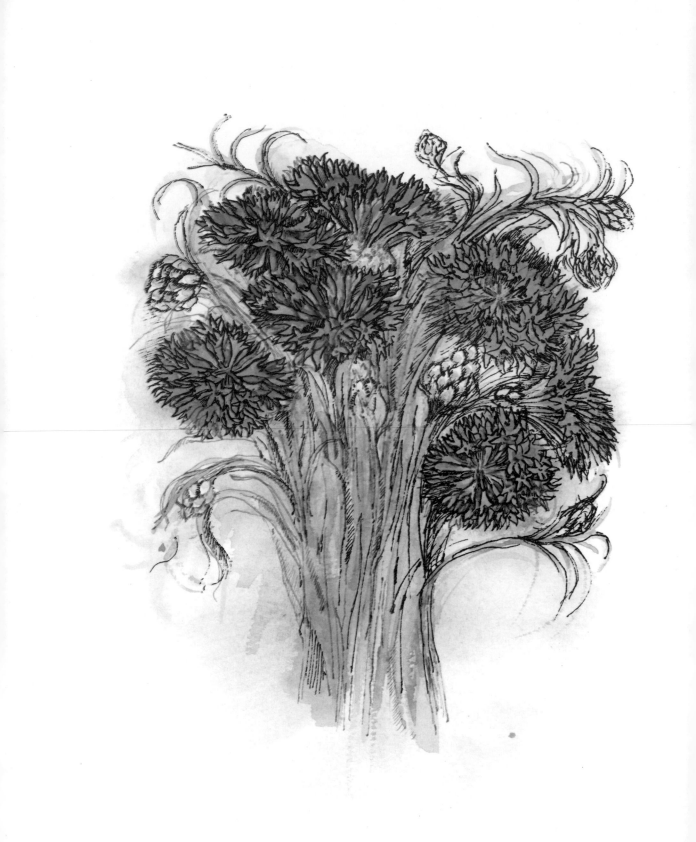

Cornflowers

Quince Lotion

Boil the quince peel as a decoction (p. 40), or juice some raw quince. Apply to the scalp several times a week.

Limeflower Lotion

Make a weak infusion of the dried flowers. Massage a little into the scalp several times a week. Limeflower stimulates the circulation of the scalp but is not astringent.

Falling Hair

There are many reasons why hair falls excessively, including poor health, poor diet, glandular imbalance and nervous tension. You should examine your state of health and your diet, and take positive steps to remedy them if they have slipped. Nervous tension creates scalp tension, impeding circulation to the scalp and starving the hair roots. Tightly pinned hair or hair pulled back tightly from the face may have the same effect. To improve the problem externally, try these two ideas:

Rosemary Massage

Make a standard infusion (p. 39), adding some thyme if you wish, and massage into the scalp regularly.

Castor Oil Massage

Warm a little oil and massage it into the scalp daily for falling hair and to encourage the growth of new hair.

Dandruff

I don't think dandruff, which is an infection of the sebaceous glands, is as common a condition as commercial advertisements would have us believe. Scaling of the scalp is quite often just skin flaking as the result of an irritating condition — perhaps through using the wrong shampoo or other hair products. Check your hair care routine. Herbs to treat dandruff are made into standard infusions (p. 39) and rubbed in daily.

Rosemary

One of the most valuable of the hair herbs. It has an antiseptic and cleansing effect on the scalp.

Nettle

A cleansing and stimulating herb, which will improve the circulation of the scalp.

Cleavers

A herb rich in silica with cooling, healing and cleansing properties.

Cider Vinegar

Use in a hair rinse after shampooing to restore the natural acid balance.

REMEDY
For Hair-Growth

Prepared For Ses, Mother of
His Majesty the King of Upper
and Lower Egypt, Teta, Deceased.

Toes-of-a-dog
Refuse-of-dates
Hoof-of-an-ass

Another Remedy to
Prevent Grey Hairs

Blood-from-the-Neck-of-
the-gabgu-bird
Put in Real Balsam and rub
therewith.

'The Papyrus Ebers'
1500 B.C.

PART VI

ABC OF HERBS & INGREDIENTS

HERBS	Oily Skin	Dry Skin	Normal Skin	Mature Skin	Sensitive Skin	Disturbed Skin	Stimulant	Soothing	Emollient	Astringent	Cleansing	Healing	Bleaching	Tonic	Hydrating
Burdock						●		●			●	●			
Chamomile	●	●	●	●	●	●		●			●	●			●
Chickweed						●			●		●	●			
Cinquefoil	●					●				●					
Clary Sage	●									●	●				
Cleavers						●					●	●			
Coltsfoot	●				●	●	●	●							
Comfrey	●	●	●	●	●	●			●	●	●	●		●	
Cowslip	●	●	●					●			●		●		
Cucumber	●	●	●	●	●				●	●			●		
Dandelion	●					●									
Elderflower	●	●	●	●	●			●	●		●	●	●		
Fennel	●	●	●	●	●			●			●			●	
Horsetail	●		●							●	●	●		●	
Houseleek	●		●			●	●			●	●				
Hyssop						●	●			●	●	●		●	
Lavender	●					●		●		●	●			●	
Lemon	●			●		●				●	●	●			
Lemon Balm	●										●				
Lemongrass	●	●				●				●	●				
Lemon Verbena	●									●					
Lettuce	●	●	●	●	●	●		●			●				
Licorice						●	●	●	●		●				
Limeflower	●		●				●	●					●		
Lovage	●					●				●	●				
Marigold	●		●			●		●		●	●				
Marjoram	●		●					●			●			●	
Marshmallow		●	●	●		●		●	●		●				
Meadowsweet						●				●	●		●		
Mint	●		●				●			●	●				
Nettle	●	●	●			●			●					●	
Orange Flower	●	●	●	●	●				●						●
Pansy						●		●	●		●				
Parsley	●					●				●					
Plantain						●	●			●	●				
Potato						●		●			●				
Red Clover						●					●				
Rose	●	●	●	●	●					●	●				●
Rosemary	●	●	●			●	●			●	●			●	
Sage	●					●	●			●	●				
Southernwood	●					●	●				●				
Summer Savory	●	●				●									
Thyme		●				●	●				●			●	
Violet	●	●	●	●	●	●		●			●	●			
Wych Hazel	●					●				●					
Yarrow	●					●				●	●	●			

Alfalfa   (MEDICAGO SATIVA)

Alfalfa is also known as lucerne, a cattle fodder. It is rich in vitamins
and minerals so is a good general tonic to boost the whole system. Buy
the dried leaves from the health shop, or grow your own from seed in
your herb garden if you want to use it fresh. It may be eaten raw in
salads or made into a tea.

Originally alfalfa grew in Asia Minor and the name comes from
the Arabic *alfacfacah* which means "best feed" (especially for horses). It
has been grown for food longer than any other known plant. It was
introduced into Greece as a horse fodder in the fourth century B.C.
and later was grown extensively by the Romans, who took it to the
rest of Europe. Alfalfa is now cultivated in many parts of the world.

Almond Meal   (PRUNUS AMYGDALUS-DULCIS)

Sweet almonds are ground up into a meal which can be used as a
facial scrub for very oily, unclean skin with blackheads. As it is fairly
abrasive rub it on gently.

Milk made from almond meal is healing, softening and slightly
astringent. It must be kept refrigerated as it goes bad quite soon when
left at room temperature. Almond milk has been used in natural
cosmetics for many generations, and is included in recipes for toners
and lotions. To make almond milk, refer to Almond Milk Toning
Lotion on page 54.

Almond Oil

A bland, essential oil expressed from the kernel of the sweet almond.
Almond oil has long been known as a reliable beautifier. Apply to dry
skin at night, smoothing into the face and neck. Leave ten to twenty
minutes, then blot off any excess with tissues, leaving a fine protective
film on the skin.

This seems to reduce the red veins in sensitive skin, softening it
and making it appear thicker and creamier. The almond tree grew
originally in Persia, Asia Minor and North Africa. Almond oil has
long been known for flavouring and scenting and is still used in
perfumery. It has been an ingredient of toilet preparations for many
centuries.

Anhydrous Lanolin

This is pure lanolin from the wool of the sheep, and is a stiff yellow
grease. It is said to be closely related to the oil produced by the

sebaceous glands in human skin, which makes it an effective lubricant and moisturiser. It has the ability to absorb large amounts of water or herbal infusion or juice, so it holds water to the skin.

To become absorbent it needs to be heated and melted. However, it is possible to make cold, hard lanolin emulsify by the addition of anything with an alcohol base, or anything acid. For example, the former could be tincture of benzoin or distilled wych hazel, the latter could be lemon juice or cider vinegar. Wool fat was used to make cosmetic unguents in the times of the ancient Greeks and Romans.

Aniseed   (PIMPINELLA ANISUM)

A member of the Umbelliferae family, with feathery leaves, the plant grows about 45 cm (18 in) high, and bears umbels of creamy-white flowers. The seed made into a tea is tonic and digestive, as well as being helpful for insomnia. Aniseed is thought to have grown originally in Egypt and Asia Minor, but is now cultivated in many parts of the world.

Anise was widely used in ancient times by the Egyptians, Greeks, Cretans and people of Asia Minor as a culinary and medicinal herb. The Romans made it into a perfume, a use which was also popular in Britain in the fourteenth century.

Apple Cider Vinegar

Apple cider vinegar must always be diluted before applying to the skin or hair, in the ratio of one teaspoon of vinegar to two tablespoons of water. Vinegar restores the acid mantle to the skin so helping to keep it in a healthy condition. On the one hand it balances up oiliness, while on the other it is valuable for dry skin which it softens while reducing flakiness. Vinegar is well-known as a hair rinse which restores acid balance to the hair after shampooing, leaving it soft and shining. It is invigorating and restorative to the body when used as a pre-bath rub or a body lotion, and is an effective deodorant.

The history of vinegar is as old as that of wine, as vinegar is in effect a wine that has gone sour. I must hasten to add that for many centuries the making of a good vinegar has been as much an art as the making of a good wine. Cider vinegar is obviously made from apples, while white wine vinegar, which may be used as a substitute, is made from grapes. Other vinegars such as malt vinegar, which is made from barley and oats, and distilled vinegar, which is made from industrial alcohol, are not suitable for cosmetic use. Vinegar has been used in cosmetic preparations since ancient times, and spirit of vinegar was reputedly one of the ingredients of the original cold cream made about the first century A.D.

Apricot Oil

Apricot kernel oil has similar attributes to almond oil so can be substituted for the latter if almond oil does not suit your skin. Apricot oil is colourless, odourless, and very light on the skin, while being very emollient. It is a delightful oil to use as a night lotion to protect the face and neck from dehydration, and is ideal as a body rub after body brushing (see p. 97).

Apricot kernel oil can be toxic when taken internally. However, there is no proof that its external use constitutes any danger, and I have used it often with benefit to the skin. Almond oil may be substituted for it in lotions, if preferred.

The apricot may have originated in China, although some consider it to be a native of the Caucasus and Armenia. It reached Europe about the time of Alexander the Great who lived in the fourth century B.C. The oil has been known and used since ancient times.

Arrowroot (MARANTA ARUNDINACEAE, etc.)

The white, powdered starch of dried arrowroot is soothing to the skin, particularly when made into a gel, although it may be also applied as a powder. It originated in South America where it was utilised by the Indians. Arrowroot has been used in England for about two hundred years.

Basil (OCIMUM BASILICUM)

This is sweet basil, a green-leafed annual, but there are other varieties — bush basil, and opal basil which has purple leaves. Basil originated in India where it is revered as a sacred plant. It was used throughout Asia Minor and Greece in ancient times, and came into general cultivation in domestic gardens in England in the sixteenth century. Culpeper, in the seventeenth century, included it in his Herbal. On the Continent it was used as a scent.

If you haven't smelt the spicy aroma of the basil plant on a hot sunny day, you've missed a delightful experience. Add some of its leaves, fresh or dried, to borage to make a relaxing tea.

Bay (LAURUS NOBILIS)

The sweet bay tree with aromatic leaves is better known for its culinary uses. It is a tree which can grow rather large in Australia, but which may be kept to smaller proportions by growing it in an ornamental tub. The leaves included in herb pillows are an old remedy against insomnia.

The bay tree is a native of the Mediterranean. Bay leaves are the laurel wreaths of honour, first used by the ancient Greeks and later by the Romans. Traditionally bay was used as a strewing herb because of its scented leaves. Medicinally it has been used as far back as the ancient Greeks, who extolled its qualities, and this use continued throughout the following centuries.

Beeswax

White beeswax is non-toxic to the skin. It has been used traditionally as an emulsifier and a binder in cosmetic creams and lip salves. It is insoluble in water. The use of beeswax in cosmetics is reputed to go back to the time of the ancient Greeks, when the first cold cream is said to have been invented.

Benzoin (SIMPLEX)

Benzoin is a reddish-brown aromatic balsam from a Javanese tree, and it can be used as a preservative in home-made cosmetics. Buy it at the chemist. It is useful for emulsifying pure wool fat (anhydrous lanolin) when making creams, when you don't want to heat the lanolin to melt it. Benzoin has a toning effect on the skin which was known to Arabian women centuries ago. It was used in perfumery as well as medicine.

Borage (BORAGO OFFICINALIS)

A herb with prickly leaves and pretty blue or pink flowers, borage sprawls across the garden, self-seeding prolifically. The leaves may be made into a standard infusion (p. 39) and used to bathe the eyes. It makes a gently relaxing tea and is a tonic and anti-inflammatory herb.

Borage originated in Asia Minor, but has become common in many other parts of the world. Its use was recorded by the ancient Greeks and Romans in medicine and in drinks.

Burdock (ARCTIUM LAPPA)

A medicinal plant, though a banned weed in many places because of the burr which spoils the fleece of sheep. It is not a true dock but a member of the Compositae family. The root is the part used cosmetically, being soothing and cleansing to irritated skin when made into a decoction (p. 40). This herb can be used in the bath or for the hair.

Burdock grew extensively throughout Europe and Central and Northern China. Historically the knowledge and use of burdock goes back to the ancient Greeks. Herbalists throughout the centuries since then have written of its properties, including its benefit for healing irritated skin conditions. Traditionally it has a long usage in China.

Buttermilk

Buttermilk is a by-product of buttermaking. Be sure to get the real churned variety. It is soothing, slightly acid and astringent, and whitening. It is excellent for any type of skin, and is especially useful during the heat of the summer when the skin needs cooling. To restore the acid balance of the skin when it appears dull and lifeless, use Buttermilk Toner (p. 53). The history of butter-making goes back to biblical times, and buttermilk has been a folk remedy for the skin for centuries.

Calendula

See Marigold.

Castor Oil

Castor oil, obtained from the castor bean, is soothing to the skin, and encourages healthy hair. It has remarkable drawing powers when applied to the skin and may be used cosmetically as well as medically.

The castor-oil plant was originally an African shrub but is grown in many countries. In medicine and perfumery, castor oil replaced a substance called castor which was obtained from the beaver. As the fresh berries of the castor-oil plant are very poisonous, it would be unwise to try to grow it.

Catmint   (NEPETA CATARIA)

A bush with scented leaves and tiny pale lavender flowers, beloved by cats for its medicinal properties. The leaves make a delightful, nerve-soothing, relaxing tea. Catmint is a hair herb, adding shine and promoting growth. It was known to early herbalists who no doubt were made aware of its properties by observing cats and other animals eating it medicinally. The seventeenth century herbalist, Culpeper, mentions its use to wash the head to take away scabs.

Chamomile   (MATRICARIA CHAMOMILLA)

This is German chamomile, a small feathery annual bearing white-petalled daisy flowers with large yellow centres. Chamomile flowers are among the most valuable of all the cosmetic herbs and are suitable for use on any part of the body. Made into an infusion for the face they are soothing and strengthening to the tissues. In shampoos or hair rinses they are lightening to the hair, thus especially good for blondes.

Taken as a tea chamomile is calming and relaxing. Chamomile originated in Europe and there are two varieties, Roman, a perennial, and German, an annual, with very similar properties. Both have a long history of use medically. German chamomile was praised by the ancient Egyptians and the Greeks. Culpeper, the English seventeenth century herbalist, tells us that an oil made from the flowers of Roman chamomile was used to anoint the body against agues and stiff joints, and that a decoction was used as a bath herb. German chamomile probably grew in Britain before Roman times and its cosmetic uses have been known for centuries.

Chickweed   (STELLARIA MEDIA)

A soft-leaved sprawling plant with tiny white flowers, chickweed grows close to the ground in weed patches, or in the paddocks.

How wasteful we are with the bounteous plants nature has given us. The despised chickweed is wonderfully healing to the skin, and is an emollient, so soothes irritated tissue. It can be used for any skin irritations. Fresh leaves can be crushed and applied directly, or they can be made into an ointment which is soothing and healing for chapped lips. It is a facial and a bath herb.

Chickweed grows wild all over the world and has been used by herbalists for centuries. Three hundred years ago, Culpeper described its use as a facial herb for any sort of skin irritation.

Cider Vinegar

See Apple Cider Vinegar.

Cinquefoil   (POTENTILLA REPTANS)

This is the "five-fingered plant", with leaves divided into five leaflets.
Use the leaves to make an infusion which is astringent to the skin
when added to the bath. It may be used on the face.

Europe is the natural habitat of cinquefoil. Culpeper describes it
as an anti-inflammatory herb for use on the skin as well as internally.
Cinquefoil was also well-known to the Greeks as a medicinal herb.

Clary Sage   (SALVIA SCLAREA)

A biennial plant of the sage family, with characteristic rough greyish-
green leaves, clary sage is obtainable at herb nurseries. The oil is a
fixative for perfumes as it is a herb which blends well with other
herbal scents. The leaves are the part used, in the bath or as a facial
lotion. The seeds were once used to make an eye lotion.

Clary sage grew originally in eastern Europe, and was taken
from there to other Continental countries. It grew in English gardens
in the seventeenth century and was described by the herbalist
Culpeper as "our ordinary garden clary". He mentions its drawing and
healing properties when applied to the skin.

Cleavers   (GALIUM APARINE)

A climbing plant with small spiky leaves, sometimes called clivers. The
leaves are the part of the herb used. Cleavers is traditionally a
deodorant herb, but is also cleansing for blemished skin. The natural
habitat of cleavers is Europe, and it has tangled the hedgerows of
Britain since time immemorial. It has been commonly known for many
centuries as healing and cleansing to the skin.

Cocoa Butter   (THEOBROMA OIL)

A solid fat from the roasted seeds of the cocoa plant which melts at
skin temperature and is very emollient and lubricant. Cocoa is
indigenous to South America and the first beans were brought to
Europe by Columbus. The beans are ground between heavy heated
rollers to melt the fat and squeeze it out. This procedure is mentioned
as early as 1753.

Coconut Oil

Coconut oil is a white, semi-solid saturated fat. It is a good lubricant for the hair and the body. A saponified version of coconut oil is sold at health shops under various brand names, being described as a bio-degradable, concentrated detergent free of additives, dyes or perfumes. Cosmetically this saponified coconut oil is useful in shampoos or the bath. The coconut palm is found in all tropical regions, and is known to have grown in tropical Asia and Malaysia since prehistoric times. Coconut oil has a long history of use in these areas.

Coltsfoot (TUSSILAGO FARFARA)

Named after the large hoof-shaped leaves which grow along the creeping rootstock. Colstfoot is emollient as well as being an astringent. It is very soothing for any inflammation of the skin and is particularly useful in the treatment of thread veins. Use the dried leaves for the face and the eyes.

Coltsfoot grows naturally in Europe, parts of India and Persia. It has a very ancient tradition as an anti-inflammatory herb internally and for skin eruptions. It is included in Culpeper's seventeenth century herbal.

Comfrey (SYMPHYTUM OFFICINALE)

A perennial plant of the borage family, comfrey has very long, hairy leaves growing from the central root. Comfrey is a cell regenerative — a useful property in cosmetics. It is one of those beautifully balanced herbs, being both astringent and emollient. Comfrey is used cosmetically wherever dryness is a problem. The fresh or dried root is the most potent part of the plant, although the leaves are also useful. A herb suitable for the face, the eyes, the hair and the bath.

Comfrey originally grew in Europe and parts of Asia. There are many varieties other than the *officinale*, the Caucasian and Russian probably being the most popular. Comfrey has been used curatively since the time of the ancient Greeks. Culpeper describes its healing properties for the skin. Ninon de Lenclos, the seventeenth century French beauty, is reputed to have included comfrey among the herbs she used to keep her skin lovely.

Cornflower (CENTAUREA CYANUS)

You may be surprised to know that the lovely blue cornflower that brightens your flower gardens has herbal properties. Gather the blue flowers to make a nerve-soothing tea for internal use, or to be applied externally to take the sting and itch out of insect bites. Cornflower infusion may be used for the eyes.

Cornflowers grow wild, particularly in the cornfields throughout Europe. It is mentioned in the literature of the ancient Greeks and Romans although apparently not in their medical writings. The cooling properties of the cornflower are described by Parkinson, a seventeenth century herbalist and apothecary. Its use for the eyes is written about in the early eighteenth century, and many years ago the French made an eyewash, *Eau de Casselunette*, from cornflowers.

Cowslip (PRIMULA VERIS)

The true cowslip, the wild flower of the springtime woods and pastures of England, is available at herbal nurseries in other countries of the world, including Australia. Its flower is a fragrant pale yellow, unlike the garden variety which has a pink edging to the petals. The petals of the flowers are the part used herbally. Made into tea they are sedative and nerve-soothing. The infusion is used externally to cleanse the skin. It is helpful to dry skin when incorporated in lotions and creams, and is known both as a facial and a bath herb.

Cowslip grows wild throughout Britain and Europe. Its use as a sedative goes back to ancient times, and there are many references in early writings to its efficacy as a beauty restorative. Culpeper describes the use of the flowers to take away spots, wrinkles, sunburn and freckles. The other seventeenth century herbalist and apothecary, John Parkinson, mentions it for the same properties.

Cucumber (CUCUMIS SATIVUS)

Cucumber is cooling and gently astringent to the skin. Put through the juice extractor, it makes a delightful lotion for the hot weather. Cucumber juice is gently bleaching for freckles, and helps prevent sunburn. Used in lotions and creams it is soothing and softening to the skin.

The cucumber probably originated in India where it has been grown for at least three thousand years. It found its way to Europe to be used by the ancient Greeks and Romans. It seems the cucumber was rather reluctantly included in salads in the sixteenth century in England after being suitably "drowned" in wine. In the *Complete Herbal* (1653), Culpeper describes its use cosmetically to cleanse and cool the face and says "it is also excellent good for sun-burning, freckles, and morphew [scurf or scaly skin]."

Dandelion   (TARAXACUM OFFICINALE)

Dandelion has oblong irregularly indented leaves, and sends up single flower stems each of which bears a simple yellow flower. It is tonic and cleansing to the body and the face. The flowers and the leaves may be used cosmetically.

Dandelion grows wild throughout most of the world. Its properties are mentioned in early Arabian medical books. In the seventeenth century Culpeper describes its use as a cleansing wash for the skin where there are sores.

Dill   (PEUCEDANUM or ANETHUM GRAVEOLENS)

A delicately flavoured, fragrant annual plant of the parsley family. Both the seeds and the leaves may be used. Usually regarded as a culinary herb or for the digestion, dill also has properties which are strengthening to the fingernails.

Dill grew wild in the Mediterranean countries and southern Russia. Its medical use is recorded as far back as the ancient Egyptians. The Greeks and Romans enjoyed it as a perfume and incense.

Distilled Water

Distilled water is purified water obtainable from the chemist. It should be used in all creams and lotions to keep them as pure and uncontaminated as possible, thus preventing too rapid deterioration. Rainwater is not really pure, though may be used if necessary.

Elderflower   (SAMBUCUS NIGRA)

The creamy-white clusters of flowers of the elderberry tree. Elderflower water has been used for generations to keep the complexion soft and white. It is one of the most useful cosmetic herbs, because it tones and protects the skin. Elderflower may be used on any part of the body.

The elder tree is native to Britain and Europe. The reputation of the berries as a hair-dye goes back to the Romans, and is mentioned by Culpeper, who also extols the flowers cosmetically "to clean the skin from sunburning, freckles, morphew [scurf or scaly skin] and the like".

Emollient

An emollient is soothing and softening to the skin.

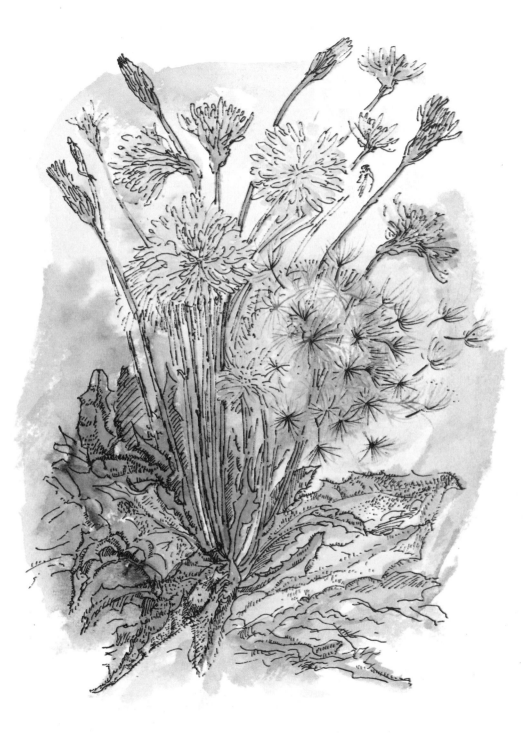

Dandelions

Eucalyptus Oil

Probably the most universally known native Australian medical or cosmetic product, eucalyptus oil is extracted from the leaves of eucalyptus trees. It is useful applied externally as a muscle relaxant.

Fennel   (FOENICULUM VULGARE)

Wild fennel has become a hardy weed in many parts of Australia and may be seen beside many roads, flourishing its characteristic tall green stems, feathery leaves and umbels of yellow flowers. Fennel is a skin tonic with strengthening qualities. It is traditionally an eye and facial herb. The seeds or the leaves are the part used cosmetically.

Fennel is native to Europe and Britain, while another variety grows wild in Syria. Its uses were known to the ancient Chinese, Indians, Egyptians, Greeks and Romans and it was included in many Roman medicines. The Anglo-Saxons used fennel and its popularity did not diminish through the centuries. It appears in herbal writings in the fourteenth, sixteenth and seventeenth centuries. Its use as an eye herb goes back to Pliny, and is recommended by the physician and herbalist Culpeper.

Flax   (LINUM USITATISSIMUM)

Flax is the blue-flowered linseed plant. Flaxseed is highly emollient, and may be used as a mucilagen in cosmetics. It is soothing to the skin, but not as healing as quince seed gel. To make flaxseed gel, simmer one cup of seed with three cups of water until thick. Strain and thin as required.

Flax is cultivated throughout many parts of the world for the oil from its seeds and the fibre from its stalks. It is not known in a wild state. Its medicinal uses and as a fibre for linen go back to the ancient Egyptians, and have a continuous history up to the present day. Its emollient properties were described by Culpeper.

Glycerin

A sweet tasting, sticky fluid obtained by adding alkali to fats or oils, usually a by-product of soap making. It is a humectant, absorbing moisture from the air. Another characteristic is its ability to facilitate the spreading of other ingredients with which it is mixed. Glycerin was first isolated by a Swedish chemist in 1779, using olive oil and lead oxide. It was named glycerin in 1813.

Honey

Honey hydrates dry or mature skin, and has softening and healing properties. It is a natural antiseptic. Honey makes a cleansing facial rub when added to oils, lotions or creams. It is very healing when made into a lip salve. The use of honey cosmetically goes back to very ancient times. It was included in herbal mixtures for applying to the skin in early Greek recipes, and its use has continued down through the centuries.

Hops (HUMULUS LUPULUS)

Hops have been known and used through the ages to soothe the nerves and induce sleep. They are the cone-like fruit borne on a perennial climbing vine. Hops are native to European countries with temperate climates. They were once commonly sold as a tea. English gardeners became interested in growing them for beer in the sixteenth century. Their medicinal properties were described in the following century by Nicholas Culpeper.

Horsetail (EQUISETUM ARVENSE)

A very ancient non-flowering perennial plant growing up to over half a metre (two feet) high from creeping rhizomes, horsetail has no leaves, just green spiky shoots which are the part used herbally. Horsetail is rich in silica and is a skin and nail tonic. It may be used on the face, and will restore skin tone after an illness. There are many species of horsetail growing throughout the world, including China, where it is also used medicinally. The Romans knew of and recommended its tonic properties. Its use as a skin cleanser and healer is described by Culpepper.

Houseleek (SEMPERVIVUM TECTORUM)

Houseleek is an astringent and cooling herb, succulent in appearance, with fleshy grey-green leaves growing in rosettes, with pink flowers borne on erect round stems covered with small scale-like leaves. It grows in many old gardens and is sometimes called hen-and-chickens. The leaves are the part used cosmetically, for the face.

Houseleek originated in the Greek islands and Europe, with related varieties growing in Africa and China. It has been regarded since ancient times as a powerful and protective herb and was grown on rooftops in China and Europe to keep thunder and lightning from the houses. Ancient Greek herbalists recommended houseleek for its cooling and healing properties for the skin and the eyes. Culpeper also mentions these uses. Houseleek is reputed to be one of the main cosmetic herbs used by the famous French beauty of the seventeenth century, Ninon de Lenclos.

Hydrate

To hydrate is to maintain the normal fluid in the skin.

Hydrating herbs are roses (petals, leaves and hips), chamomile flowers and orange blossoms. Other natural moisturisers are honey, lanolin and glycerin.

Hyssop   (HYSSOPUS OFFICINALIS)

A small bush with branchy stems bearing dark green leaves and tiny blue flowers, hyssop has a centuries-old reputation as a cleansing and healing herb. It is astringent and tonic, being stimulating to the skin and body when added to the bath. The leaves and the flowers are used.

Hyssop is a native of central and southern Europe. It was known and used medically by ancient Greek physicians. Centuries later the herbalist Culpeper suggests its use externally: "boiled with wine, it is good to wash inflammations, and takes away the blue and black marks that come by strokes, bruises and falls, if applied with warm water". Culpeper says too that fresh bruised leaves will quickly heal cuts or wounds.

Irish Moss   (CHONDRUS CRISPUS)

This is a seaweed which looks like moss. It is also known as carrageen. It is a soothing emollient in cosmetics, and acts as a stabiliser and emulsifier in creams. Seaweeds or sea plants have commonly been used by man for many centuries. Irish moss is found on the sea coasts of Europe and the U.S.A.

Kaolin

A fine white clay used in making various products including fine porcelain, paper, cloth, paint and soap. It is obtainable from the chemist.

Lanolin

See Anhydrous Lanolin.

Lavender   (LAVANDULA OFFICINALIS)

English lavender has more fragrance than the French variety.
Lavender is a herb which has the opposing qualities of being both a
stimulant and a sedative. Taken internally as a tea or sniffed as dried
flowers, its effect is sedating to the nerves. Used externally, it is
stimulating and antiseptic, hence its use as a skin tonic for oily skin
and pimples. It may be used on the face or in the bath as in infusion.
Herbs it blends well with are rosemary, comfrey and rose. Lavender oil
is good for the hair.

Lavender came originally from the Mediterranean countries,
where it was used and enjoyed by the ancient Greeks and Romans as
an aromatic bath herb, and to allay stiffness. English lavender was not
cultivated in England until about the sixteenth century, but was
imported dried prior to that date. It was popular as a sweet washing
water for the body and as a sedative in herb pillows or cushions. The
sedating properties of its aroma are described by Culpeper. It is
reputed to be one of the herbs used by the seventeenth century
French beauty Ninon de Lenclos for her skin care.

Lecithin

Lecithin is a natural emulsifier. Liquid lecithin is made from the soy
bean and is available at health shops.

Lemon   (CITRUS LIMON)

The lemon is the most useful fruit for cosmetic purposes. The juice is
acid so counteracts the alkalinity of soaps and shampoos, hence
combating chapping and dryness. It has a long traditional use as a
skin bleach. Lemon juice makes lanolin (wool fat) emulsify without
needing to melt it, so is useful in making cosmetic creams. A warm
lemon drink at bedtime often helps promote a restful sleep.

The lemon was probably a native of India or the Middle East.
Its antiseptic properties have been known since ancient times, and it
was used medicinally by the Greeks. Cosmetically it is mentioned as
an ingredient in *The Toilet of Flora*, a herbal skin-care book published
in London in 1775.

Lemon Balm   (MELISSA OFFICINALIS)

Lemon balm is a perennial bush growing about half a metre (two feet)
high, with a delightful spicy-lemon fragrance. Taken as a herbal tea it
has a calming effect on the stomach and nerves. The leaves are the

part to use, for the face, the hair or in the bath. A cleansing and antiseptic herb.

Lemon balm grew originally in the Middle East and southern Europe, and was probably taken to Britain by the Romans. Balm tea has been made for many centuries. Its use for cleansing the skin was described in the seventeenth century by Nicholas Culpeper, who also mentions that balm was extolled by the Arabians.

Lemongrass   (CYMBOPOGON CITRATUS)

Lemongrass is a tropical grass which grows readily in most parts of Australia, or can be obtained dried from health shops. It is rich in vitamin A. It is used cosmetically to normalise the sebaceous or oil glands. The rather stiff, grass-like leaves are the part of the plant used for the face, the bath or the hair.

There are two main varieties of lemongrass which grow in tropical areas, one in the West Indies, and the other in the East Indies, both of which have been used for generations by the indigenous people.

Lemon Verbena   (ALOYSIA CITRIODORA or HIPPIA CITRIODORA)

A delightful garden shrub. It has strongly perfumed leaves which are fragrant with the scent of lemon. The leaves can be made into a relaxing and cooling tea. Lemon verbena is an astringent herb used for the hair and the skin around the eyes.

Lemon verbena is a native of South America and was not introduced into England until the late eighteenth century. It soon became popular for use in colognes, teas and herb pillows.

Lettuce   (LACTUCA SATIVA)

This is the domestic or garden lettuce of which there are several interesting varieties currently available. A wild variety also exists. Of the domestic types, I find the dainty loose-leafed Mignonettes, or the upright Cos, far better than the tight-leaved Iceberg type. Cosmetically the juice of the lettuce is soothing to the skin, when used on the face or in the bath.

Lettuce is cultivated all over the world and its place of origin is uncertain. Its origins go back to ancient times, and its sedative effect when used internally has been known since then. According to the seventeenth century herbalist, Culpeper, "The juice mixed or boiled with oil of roses, applied to the forehead and temples, procures sleep . . . ."

Licorice (GLYCYRRHIZA GLABRA)

A perennial shrub which grows up to one and a quarter metres (four feet), bearing dark green leaves and spikes of yellow-white or purple flowers. The powdered root of the licorice is used in cosmetics, because it reduces inflammation and soothes the skin. It may be used on the face. Licorice makes an astringent for the gums and adds flavour to toothpowder.

Licorice probably originated in the East, gradually spreading through central Asia to Europe and north Africa. The ancient Chinese used it medicinally, as did the Egyptians, Assyrians, Sumerians, Babylonians and Hindus. The Greeks and Romans extolled its properties.

Limeflowers (TILIA EUROPAEA)

Limeflowers are borne on the lime or linden tree, and have a fragrant scent. Cosmetically they are used on the face to bleach and to stimulate the skin. Made into a tea, they are a refreshing and nerve soothing drink.

Linden trees grew originally in Europe and Britain and mention of them goes back to classical times.

Lovage (LEVISTICUM OFFICINALE)

Lovage, which has a celery-like leaf and flavour, is a perennial which will grow up to one and a half metres (five feet) high. Traditionally it has a deodorant effect on the skin when added to the bath or applied under the arms. The leaves are the part of the plant used.

Lovage is a native of the Mediterranean countries and was used by the ancient Romans and Greeks for its medicinal and antiseptic qualities, as well as cosmetically. It was cultivated in England in the fourteenth century. The seventeenth century herbalist Culpeper says that it removes spots and freckles from the face.

Marigold (CALENDULA OFFICINALIS)

The calendula is the flat petalled English or pot marigold, and the orange-coloured flower is the one used herbally. It is remarkably healing to the skin when used on the face or in the bath.

It may have come originally from India, but the marigold is now regarded as a native of southern Europe. Its healing properties were known to the Romans and the Arabs, but it was not well-known in

Europe until some centuries later. All the English herbal writers of the sixteenth, seventeenth and eighteenth centuries recommended it. It was known for use cosmetically as a dye to make the hair yellow. Marigold Water was made in Tudor times and used as a perfume.

Marjoram   (ORIGANUM VULGARE)

Sweet marjoram, with its small round leaves and knots of greenish-white flowers, is usually regarded as a culinary herb, but it does have medicinal and cosmetic uses also. It is a tonic to the skin and calming to the body when added to a bath.

There are several varieties of marjoram which originated in Mediterranean countries. It has a long history of use, being included in perfumes by the Greeks and Romans. It has been popular for centuries in England because of its aromatic qualities which were used in sweet washing waters, sweet bags or sachets, and pillows.

Marshmallow   (ALTHAEA OFFICINALIS)

A shrub-like plant with large grey-green leaves and clusters of pink flowers. A decoction of the root of the marshmallow is healing and emollient because it contains much mucilage. It is combined with other herbs such as comfrey, rose or lily-bulbs in lotions and creams to moisturise the skin. Suitable for the face, the body and the hair. The leaves may also be used.

Although marshmallow is a native of Europe it may have been brought originally from China. It was well known to the ancient Greeks and Romans for its healing qualities. It has a history of usage through the succeeding centuries, and was included in English herbals of the seventeenth century where its soothing and healing properties for the skin are mentioned.

Meadowsweet   (FILIPENDULA ULMARIA)

A herb of the English meadows producing creamy, sweetly scented flowers. Meadowsweet is available at herb nurseries. Delightful for scenting the skin as well as being a complexion tonic.

Europe is the natural habitat of the meadowsweet although it also grows wild in parts of Asia. Medicinally it is mentioned in English herbals of the sixteenth and seventeenth centuries, where its healing qualities, both internally and externally, are recommended. Meadowsweet has been valued for centuries for its sweet fragrance, and was commonly used as a strewing herb and added to drinks.

Mignonette   (RESEDA ODORATA)

Garden mignonette, which bears sweetly smelling yellowish-green flowers, is charming rather than showy in the flower garden. There is a wild variety (*Reseda lutea*). Mignonette is a relaxing and sleep-inducing herb suitable for use in herb pillows.

This herb is a native of Egypt. It became popular in France and was sent from there to England in 1742, where it was quickly appreciated for its sweet scent and sedative properties. Mignonette was used medicinally in Roman times.

Mint   (MENTHA spp.)

Used externally, mint is a stimulant. Internally it soothes the stomach. There are many kinds of mint which may be used on their own or combined with other herbs for cosmetics. Spearmint and peppermint (p. 190) are used for the face. Any of the mints, including applemint and eau-de-cologne mint, are used for bathing. The leaves are the part used.

Mint is cultivated all over the world and there are many varieties. It has been known and used since ancient times. The Greeks made it into perfume for particular use on the arms; and the Egyptians, Romans and Arabs used it in many ways for its aromatic qualities. It was included in English herbals.

Moisturiser

A moisturiser holds water to the skin, so helping it retain its natural moisture and keeping it soft and supple.

Mucilage

A mucilage is soothing to the skin and is made by combining the sticky or gelatinous parts of plants with water. Mucilages can be made from marshmallow or comfrey roots, Irish moss, quince or flax seeds, to name a few examples.

Nettle   (URTICA DIOICA)

The English stinging nettle is horribly irritant to the skin when fresh, but quite safe to touch when dried. It is a very medicinal herb. The leaves are the part of the plant used. A skin and hair tonic and stimulant, nettle encourages circulation.

The nettle is regarded as native to Britain, but grows throughout many parts of the world. Originally it may have been brought there by the Romans. It has been used for tonic purposes and to encourage circulation since ancient times. The seventeenth century herbalist Culpeper says it is good to rub into "cold and benumbed members". He recommends it too as a wash to cleanse the skin.

Oats   (AVENA SATIVA)

Oatmeal is soothing and healing to the skin. Oatmeal flour is very useful as a substitute for soap when made into bath bags with the addition of various herbs. It may be used as a facial cleanser, mask, softener or nourisher. Steel-cut oats are used as a gentle toner and mask.

Oats were probably native to Asia but have been cultivated for many centuries elsewhere. They have long been regarded as a valuable cosmetic aid. Culpeper says, "The meal of oats boiled with vinegar and applied, takes away freckles and spots in the face and other parts of the body."

Oils

Use only cold-pressed vegetable and nut oils, without preservatives, anti-oxidants or other additives. I don't use mineral oil, which is liquid paraffin, as it leaches vitamins out of the body.

Oils can be used as cleansers for dry or sensitive skins, as well as soothers, nourishers and protecters. Oils of many varieties have been used cosmetically to cleanse and lubricate the skin since ancient times.

Olive Oil

Olive oil is too thick and heavy to use in creams or lotions unless it is diluted with a lighter oil. It sits too heavily on the skin to be left on for any length of time. However, it is excellent for use as a cleanser for dry skin. Herbs may be steeped in it to make herbal oils. It is a useful emollient for the body and the hair and relaxing to muscles and nerves.

The olive is thought to have originated in Syria and moved thence through Africa to the Mediterranean countries of Europe. The olive press is said to be as old as the wine press, and the oil has been used cosmetically for the body and hair since that time.

Orange Flower   (CITRUS SINENSIS)

The white blossom of the orange tree, famed as a head circlet for brides. Orange flower water hydrates the skin, so is useful in facial lotions or rinses.

The orange is believed to have originated in central Asia, being taken thence to Mediterranean countries. Orange flower water has been used by generations internally as a digestive and sedative and externally as a cosmetic.

Orris   (IRIS FLORENTINA)

Orris is the powdered root of the dried rhizome of the Florentine iris, and is reminiscent of violets in scent. It is used as a fixative in perfumes. It is useful in toothpowders or toothpastes and gives a delightful hint of violet to bathbags.

The Florentine iris originated in Italy and Morocco. It is reputed to have been used in ancient Egypt as an ingredient of incense. Orris is valued mainly for its fragrance and was included for this reason in lubricating ointments in ancient Greece. It was used for centuries as an ingredient of toilet powders and in teeth cleaning preparations to sweeten the breath.

Pansy   (VIOLA TRICOLOR)

This is the wild pansy bearing tiny purple flowers with typical markings of white and yellow. The garden pansy is a much larger, showier plant. *Viola tricolor* or Heartsease is obtainable at herb nurseries in Australia. It is mucilaginous and emollient and very healing for any skin type, and may be used on the face or the body. The whole plant is used.

The pansy grows wild in Britain, but has been cultivated for many centuries. It was included in the English herbals of the seventeenth century where its cooling and emollient properties were recommended for skin irritations.

Parsley   (PETROSELINUM CRISPUM)

Parsley, so well-known but so often disregarded as a mere decoration or garnish for food, has many useful properties cosmetically, being cleansing and soothing. It is beneficial for the face, the eyes, the hair and as a deodorant. Use the leaves.

Parsley originated in eastern Mediterranean countries. It is mentioned in seventeenth century herbals as being useful to soothe the eyes, and to take away bruise marks from the skin.

Pennyroyal   (MENTHA PULEGIUM)

A pungent herb which makes a delightful ground cover, with its bright green leaves and spikes of lavender coloured flowers. The aromatic leaves are useful as a mouth wash or an insect repellant.

Pennyroyal is a member of the mint family, originating in Europe. Its use cosmetically was mentioned by Culpeper, who recommended it to be applied as a plaster to take away marks and spots on the face.

Peppermint (MENTHA PIPERITA)

This mint, which has very dark purplish-green leaves on reddish stems, is the type of mint most often used cosmetically. Externally it is a cooling and antiseptic herb. Internally it is warming and tonic to the digestive and nervous systems, so an infusion of peppermint makes a relaxing tea. Oil of peppermint is used as a flavouring oil in toothpaste, or to mentholate lip salve.

Peppermint was named as a separate mint species in the seventeenth century. Mint has been used in teeth-cleaning preparations for many centuries.

Photo-sensitivity

The skin may become over-sensitive to light through the application of certain substances, vegetable or chemical. Symptoms may include rashes, redness, swelling and hyper-pigmentation.

Plantain (PLANTAGO MAJOR)

Long regarded as a weed in paddocks and gardens, the plantain has been a despised herb. Plantain leaves grow in flat rosettes and are prominently veined. It bears spikes of brownish flowers clustered closely along the stem. The leaves are soothing and healing to the skin for irritated insect bites.

Plantain grows throughout the world and ancient Greek and Roman physicians recommended it medicinally. The English herbalist Culpeper also recommended it for its healing properties.

Potato (SOLANUM TUBEROSUM)

The juice of the raw potato is soothing, anti-inflammatory and reduces puffiness. It speedily reduces dark areas when applied to a bruise. It may be used on the face and the body.

The potato is a tropical plant and a native of South America, introduced into England in the sixteenth century. It was probably used as a folk remedy for many generations. The gypsies used raw potato internally to promote the curing of skin diseases.

Pumpkin Oil

A thick, dark, very healing oil, rather pungent smelling, extracted from the pumpkin seed. When used cosmetically it is better thinned with a light, bland oil such as apricot.

The pumpkin originated in America, being used by the Indians, and was unknown to Europeans until they settled the continent.

Purslane   (PORTULACA OLERACEA)

A valuable little herb which grows happily in harsh, dry conditions, and which we industriously pull out of our gardens as a weed. It has red, fleshy stems, ovate thick green leaves, and little yellow flowers. It is rich in vitamins and minerals. Use the leaves as a tonic, made into a tea, or in a salad.

Purslane grows throughout the world and has been used as a culinary herb in Asia for centuries. Its use as an anti-inflammatory herb for the skin and eyes is mentioned in seventeenth century herbals.

Quince   (PYRUS CYDONIA)

This is the large, hard yellow-skinned fruit from the quince tree. The seeds of ripe quince are the part most valuable for use in cosmetics, as they produce a thick gel when soaked or simmered. The jelly is used as a demulcent and emulsifier in lotions and creams and is very healing to the skin, as well as being an excellent setting lotion for the hair. Don't throw away the quince peel, as it can be simmered with water for use as a hair rinse.

The quince is a native of Persia, but is now grown in many countries throughout the world. The gel made from the seeds is described by the seventeenth century herbalist Culpeper. He recommends it as being cooling and healing to the mouth, the tongue and the skin. He says the boiled "down" of the quince, rubbed into the scalp, will prevent the hair from falling or restore hair to those who are bald.

Red Clover   (TRIFOLIUM PRATENSE)

One of the treats I give myself when I visit my native land, New Zealand, is to gather the sweet-smelling, honey-tasting flower heads of red clover growing in the green paddocks. When made into a tea they are soothing to the nerves and help promote sleep. An infusion is used for the hair or in the bath.

Red clover grows throughout Europe and many other countries. It was mentioned by the sixteenth century herbalist, Gerard.

Rose (ROSA spp.)

The species of rose most commonly used cosmetically are the old-fashioned Centifolia, Damascena and Gallica roses. Highly perfumed modern roses, particularly the dark red varieties, may be substituted. Rosewater hydrates the skin and is cleansing and mildly astringent. It is used on the face and the body.

The rose originated in Persia, but has been cultivated throughout Europe for many centuries. Other varieties of the rose are indigenous to China. The rose has been used since ancient times for cosmetic purposes in the form of oil or water. Oil of roses is reputedly an ingredient of the original cold cream made in ancient Greece. Every age since then has had its uses for the rose.

Culpeper says that an ointment of roses will cool and heal red pimples in the face.

Rosehip (ROSA CANINA)

The rosehip is the fruit of the rose. The old-fashioned dog-rose, which can be found growing wild along the roadsides provides the rosehips with high vitamin C content which are gathered for pharmaceutical use. Highly bred garden roses may produce large hips, but they contain little of the vitamin. To encourage a beautiful skin drink rosehip tea. Externally, the tea may be used as a compress to reduce puffiness around the eyes, or included in lotions and creams.

Rosehips have been used in the diet of many peoples for thousands of years for their flavour and fragrance as well as medicinally.

Rosemary (ROSMARINUS OFFICINALIS)

A well-known aromatic, low-growing shrub, with spiky, dark green leaves and clusters of small pale, blue flowers. Rosemary is a cleansing, stimulating and restorative herb, to be used on the body either as an infusion, or in the form of an essential oil. It is beneficial for the hair, as well as being a deodorant, a mouthwash and a bath herb. The leaves and soft twigs are used.

Rosemary originated in Mediterranean countries, and was probably introduced into Britain by the Romans. It was first mentioned in English herbals in the eleventh century. An early cosmetic use was in Queen of Hungary water, a fourteenth century recipe which was claimed to be restorative to the face and body. Rosemary is mentioned as being popular as a bath herb by Culpeper. He gives directions for distilling the oil to take away spots, marks and scars on the skin.

Sage   (SALVIA OFFICINALIS)

We tend to take this well-known herb for granted because it has been used for so many generations in the kitchen. However, do not underestimate it. Its botanical name means "health". The leaves are used. Made into a tea sage is refreshing to the palate and strengthening to the nerves. It is effective as a deodorant, a tooth polisher and whitener, for the hair, or in the bath. It is astringent.

Sage originated in Mediterranean countries, where it was considered a sacred herb by the Romans. It has been used since ancient times as a medicinal herb, being described by ancient Greek and Roman physicians and later herbalists. Sage has been a folk method of cleaning the teeth for many centuries. It is mentioned as an ingredient in a teeth-cleansing preparation in *The Toilet of Flora*, published in London in 1779.

St John's Wort   (HYPERICUM PERFORATUM)

A rather dainty-looking perennial which bears small, bright yellow flowers reminiscent of the poppy. A medicinal plant, valued mainly for its oil, which is soothing and healing. A tea made from the leaves may be taken to soothe the nerves.

St John's wort originated in Europe and India and grows wild throughout Britain, Europe and Asia. It is available in herb nurseries elsewhere. Its healing red oil has been made and used for centuries and was particularly popular in the Middle Ages as a treatment for wounds.

Southernwood   (ARTEMISIA ABROTANUM)

A pungent herb of the wormwood family, stimulating and cleansing to the hair and the body. It is shrub-like in appearance, with woody stems and feathery grey-green leaves.

Southernwood is native to southern Europe, and has been cultivated in gardens in England for about four centuries. In 1653 the herbalist Culpeper recommended it to be boiled with barley-meal to remove pimples from the face. He also claimed that the ashes of the leaves mixed with salad oil will promote hair growth. Southernwood is mentioned as a hair herb in *The Toilet of Flora*.

Summer Savory   (SATUREJA HORTENSIS)

A bushy annual herb with a delightful aroma. Taken as a tea, it is soothing to the stomach and intestines as well as quieting the nerves. Used externally in the bath it is a stimulant to the skin and body.

Savory is a native of Mediterranean countries and has been used since Roman times as a culinary herb. The seventeenth century English herbalist, Culpeper, described its medicinal uses.

Thyme   (THYMUS VULGARIS)

This is garden thyme with its tiny pungent leaves and dainty lilac flowers. Thyme is well known as a natural disinfectant and antiseptic. Thymol is the essential oil extracted from the thyme plant. Thyme is useful in toothpowders or toothpastes, mouthwashes and underarm deodorants. It may be used occasionally as a facial tonic as it is a stimulant and encourages the flow of blood to the surface of the skin.

Thyme originated in southern Europe and Asia Minor. Its fragrance has been appreciated since ancient times when it was used as a perfume by Greek and Roman men, and as an invigorating bath. Its antiseptic properties were recognised and it was used as a fumigant. During later centuries the English planted it in aromatic gardens.

Violet   (VIOLA ODORATA)

Both the fragrant purple flowers and the leaves of the violet are used cosmetically. They are soothing and cleansing to the skin as well as being gently astringent. The violet is suitable for all skin types, and may be used on the face and the body.

The violet originated in Europe where it was appreciated by the ancient Greeks and Romans for making cosmetics, perfumes, medicines and fragrant drinks and food. The ancient Britons made a violet facial lotion by steeping the flowers in goat's milk. Its popularity and use continued throughout the centuries, with violet mentioned for use in salads, sweets and cordials, perfumes, cosmetics and pillows.

Wallflower   (CHEIRANTHUS CHEIRI)

The perennial wallflower, bearing sweetly-scented yellow flowers, is perhaps better known for its inclusion in pot-pourri. The flowers have properties which are soothing to the nerves and muscles.

The wallflower was native to northern Europe and India. It was reputedly used in the cosmetic recipes of ancient times.

Wheatgerm Oil

An unsaturated fatty acid obtained from the wheat seed. A light, fine oil rich in vitamin E which is healing to the skin.

Wheat was grown in prehistoric times, probably six to seven thousand years ago. Evidence of its cultivation has been found in Europe, England, Egypt and China.

Wool Fat

See Anhydrous Lanolin.

Wych Hazel   (HAMAMELIS VIRGINIANA)

A small, deciduous tree, the bark and leaves being used. Wych hazel is an astringent and styptic herb. It is well-known as a skin freshener and refrigerant, particularly for oily skin. It will help to reduce the size of the large pores which accompany this skin type. It is also useful as an underarm deodorant. Distilled wych hazel is obtainable from the chemist.

Wych hazel is a native of America where it was used medicinally by the Indians, its most valuable use being for the skin.

Yarrow   (ACHILLEA MILLEFOLIUM)

A perennial plant with a creeping rootstock, bearing feathery green leaves and white or pink umbels of tiny flowers. Yarrow is an astringent and cleansing herb as well as being a styptic (a substance that stops bleeding). Don't use it on the face as a general wash or lotion because it may cause photosensitivity. Use it as a mouthwash and in shampoos.

Yarrow grows wild in Europe, Asia and North America. Its styptic properties have been known since ancient times when it was widely used as a wound herb.

APPENDIX: DRYING HERBS AT HOME

Correctly dried herbs have their water content eliminated while retaining the essential oils, fragrance and natural chemical composition of the plant. Before discussing harvesting and drying, I should like to make brief reference to the growing of herbs so that they are especially fragrant with a concentrated oil content. The secret is not to overfeed them. Fertilise herbs twice a year only — in the spring and at the beginning of autumn. Use natural fertilisers, such as compost, animal manure or blood and bone, rather than chemical fertilisers which cause plants to take up a great deal of water, making them much more difficult to dry.

As a general rule, herbs should be harvested just as they are coming into bloom. However, lavender and thyme are two well-known favourites which are better left until in full bloom. Pick the herbs in mid-morning on a dry day after any overnight dew has dried, but before the sun becomes too hot. Be careful to select undamaged, insect-free leaves and flowers. It should not be necessary to rinse them unless they are obviously dirty, and if you do rinse, dry them on a paper towel. Always handle the plant material carefully so as not to bruise it as this causes brown discolouration when dry.

It is essential to dry leaves and flowers in the shade away from bright sunlight, otherwise they lose oils, fragrance and colour. Indoors in a well-ventilated room or shed is ideal. Some herbs such as lavender, thyme, sage, rosemary and lemon verbena may be hung upside down in bunches to dry. Lavender dries well too, upside down in large brown paper bags. Spread rose petals, rose geranium leaves and so on in single layers in shallow boxes or baskets lined with newspaper, or make screens of curtain net or wire mesh stretched over wooden frames if you want ventilation all round the plant material.

It is necessary to have a steady temperature — between 25°C (75°F) and 30°C (85°F) — during the first 24 hours, and to turn the herbs frequently in order to reduce the moisture content quickly. For the remaining four or five days of the drying time a temperature of

20°C (68°F) is adequate. Herbs are sufficiently dry when they snap easily between the fingers.

When harvesting the roots of herbs, dig them in the autumn, wash and scrub them, then cut them lengthwise into narrow slivers. They may be strung up or spread on screens to dry in the sun or in a heated room. To gather seeds, pick the flower heads when they are fully ripe and dried on the plant. Pick them into brown paper bags and shake the seeds out of the flower heads.

Store dried herbs in dark air-tight containers. Those with cork stoppers are ideal, although glass or plastic jars with screw tops are adequate.

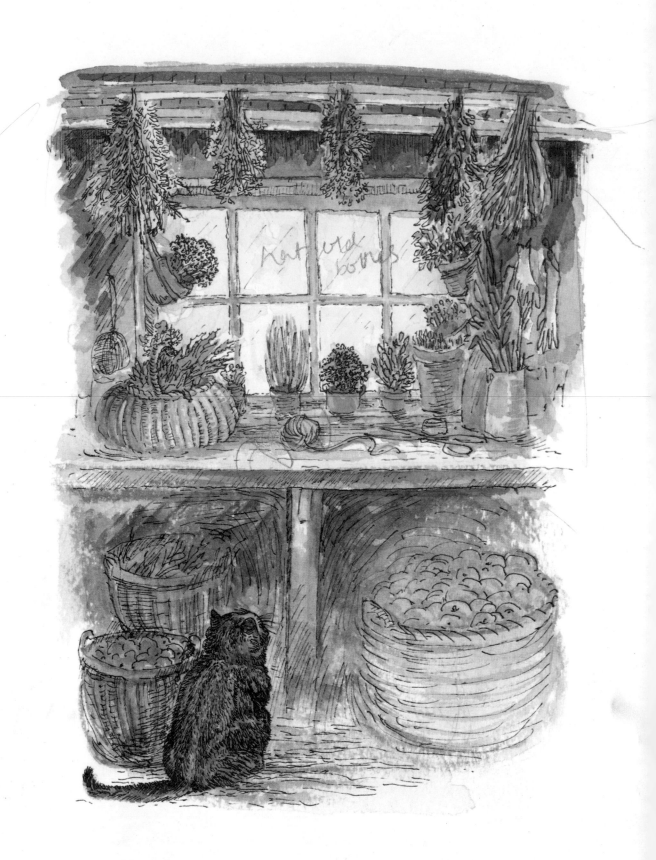

INDEX

QUOTATIONS

"A Garden of Herbs", Rohde, E.S., London, 1926.

"Culpeper's Complete Herbal", Foulsham, W., London. Wellington, 1948.

"Gerard's Herball", Gerard, G. (Marcus Woodward), Gerald Howe, London, 1927.

"How to be Beautiful", Weldon, P., Adelaide, 1913.

"Madame Cristo's Beauty Guide", Newman, E.M., Adelaide, 1923.

"Natural History", Pliny, trans Rackham H., Heinemann, London.

"Pam" A South Australian Monthly Ladies Journal, Adelaide 1923/4.

"Shopping" The Australian Housewife's Monthly Newspaper, Adelaide, 1918.

"The Greek Herbal of Dioscorides", Gunther, R.T., Hafner Publ. Co., N. York, 1959.

"The Lover's Handbook", Ovid, trans Wright, F.A., Routledge, London, 1925.

"The Magic of Herbs", Leyel, Mrs C.F., London, 1926

"The Papyrus Ebers", trans Bryan, C.T., Geoff Bles., London, 1930.

"The Toilet of Flora", trans from "La Toilette De Flora", Buc' Hoz, P.J. Murray & Nicholl, London, 1775.